Advanced Prescribing in Psychosis

The Maudsley
Guidelines on Advanced Prescribing in Psychosis

Paul Morrison

Argyll and Bute Hospital
Scotland, UK
and
Institute of Psychiatry
Psychology and Neuroscience
King's College London
London, UK

David M. Taylor

Maudsley Hospital
and
King's College London
London, UK

Phillip McGuire

Institute of Psychiatry
Psychology and Neuroscience
King's College London
London, UK

WILEY Blackwell

Registered Offices
John Wiley & Sons, Inc., 111 River Street, Hoboken, NJ 07030, USA
John Wiley & Sons Ltd, The Atrium, Southern Gate, Chichester, West Sussex, PO19 8SQ, UK

Editorial Office
111 River Street, Hoboken, NJ 07030, USA

For details of our global editorial offices, customer services, and more information about Wiley products visit us at www.wiley.com.

Wiley also publishes its books in a variety of electronic formats and by print-on-demand. Some content that appears in standard print versions of this book may not be available in other formats.

Library of Congress Cataloging-in-Publication Data

Names: Morrison, Paul, 1956– author. | Taylor, David M., 1963– author. |
    McGuire, Philip, author.
Title: The Maudsley guidelines on advanced prescribing in psychosis / Paul
    Morrison, David M. Taylor, Phillip McGuire.
Other titles: Guidelines on advanced prescribing in psychosis
Description: Hoboken, NJ : Wiley-Blackwell, 2020. | Includes
    bibliographical references and index.
Identifiers: LCCN 2019047707 (print) | LCCN 2019047708 (ebook) | ISBN
    9781119578444 (paperback) | ISBN 9781119578529 (adobe pdf) | ISBN
    9781119578437 (epub)
Subjects: MESH: Psychotic Disorders–drug therapy | Antipsychotic
    Agents–side effects | Evidence-Based Medicine | Physician-Patient
    Relations | Treatment Outcome
Classification: LCC RC483 (print) | LCC RC483 (ebook) | NLM WM 200 | DDC
    616.89/18–dc23
LC record available at https://lccn.loc.gov/2019047707
LC ebook record available at https://lccn.loc.gov/2019047708

Cover Design: Wiley

Set in 10/12pt Sabon by SPi Global, Pondicherry, India
Printed and bound by CPI Group (UK) Ltd, Croydon, CR0 4YY

C9781119578444_200624

Contents

List of tables

Preface

Prescribing guidelines proceed on the basis that all individuals with a given diagnosis suffer from an identical illness, with common underlying mechanisms. In general medicine, this is taken for granted and is not even an issue. For the treatment of psychosis, things are not so straightforward. In contrast to general medical conditions, a one-size-fits-all approach for the treatment of psychosis is unfeasible.

Psychosis can occur in various distinct psychiatric syndromes including schizophrenia, bipolar disorder, major depression and obsessive compulsive disorder. Psychotic experiences can occur in normal health but can also be a marker of serious organic pathology, for example, antibodies directed toward specific ion channels in brain tissue. Throughout the text we emphasise that the treatment of psychosis must be tailored to the needs of the individual patient.

Although classification remains problematic in psychiatry, the same is not true of psychopharmacological treatments. Over a period of 20 years or so, beginning in the early 1950s, there emerged genuinely effective medicines for major psychiatric syndromes. For the first time it was possible to provide symptomatic improvement (and not just sedation) for mania, thought disorder, delusions, hallucinations, breakdown of ego boundaries and so forth. And it became apparent, within a few years, that maintenance treatment could prevent a relapse back into psychosis and keep people out of hospital.

A range of psychopharmacological options are available for patients, with important differences between the various drugs. We adopt the strategy of comparing the upside versus the downside of each pharmaceutical. The ideal scenario is where the prescriber and the patient can weigh up the benefits versus the costs of each option and make joint decisions on treatment.

We differentiate the acute from the maintenance stage, as regards the aims of pharmacological treatment. In the acute stage, symptom relief is the priority. In the maintenance stage, the aim is to avoid relapse, which aside from further suffering, predicts a poor functional outcome. Without medication, about 80–90% of people diagnosed with bipolar disorder or schizophrenia will experience a relapse. With maintenance medication, the risk reduces to between 5% and 40%. Genuine collaboration is much more feasible in the maintenance compared to the acute stage, this being particularly notable in bipolar disorder.

There are sections on the common side effects of all widely used antipsychotic drugs, especially for clozapine, the most powerful antipsychotic. The aim is to have data close to hand for the prescriber, care coordinator, patients and their family. We incorporate a brief explanation of the molecular origin of each side effect to aid understanding and joint decision making. The ethos is that patients should be provided with accurate data to be able to make informed healthcare decisions for themselves.

In the final two sections, the emphasis shifts from the individual toward the population level and the systems in which treatment takes place. The task is to configure resources for optimum benefit at minimal cost. We introduce the principles of value-based healthcare and highlight the emergence of engineering principles in healthcare delivery systems. Both developments hold the promise of bringing the management of healthcare delivery under the scientific gaze.

When selecting a drug, it is useful to have basic, accurate data close to hand, covering the pharmacokinetics, interactions and the requisite physical health checks for each drug. We hope that psychiatrists, pharmacists and nurse prescribers will find the tables at the end of the book helpful for this purpose, even in a busy clinical setting.

Glossary

AKT	RAC-alpha serine/threonine-protein kinase	hERG	Human-ether-a-go-go-related gene
BLIP	Brief limited intermittent psychosis	HDAC	Histone deacetylase
CGI	Clinical global impression	HTT	Home treatment team
CMHT	Community mental health team	ICD10	International statistical classification of diseases 10th Edition
CNS	Central nervous system	IM	Intramuscular
CBD	Cannabidiol	LSD	Lysergic acid diethylamide
CBT	Cognitive behavioural therapy	NMDA	N-methyl-D-aspartate
CRT	Cognitive remediation therapy	NICE	National institute of Clinical Excellence
DKA	Diabetic ketoacidosis	OCD	Obsessive compulsive disorder
ECT	Electroconvulsive therapy	RCT	Randomised controlled trial
EI	Early intervention	SLAM	South London & Maudsley NHS Foundation Trust
EPSEs	Extrapyramidal side-effects		
GABA	γ-aminobutyric acid	SSRI	Selective serotonin reuptake inhibitor
GAF	Global assessment of functioning	TD	Tardive dyskinesia
GLP-1	Glucagon-like peptide-1	THC	delta-9-tetrahydrocannabinol
GSK3β	Glycogen synthase kinase 3β	UDS	Urine drug screen

Acknowledgments

We thank the following people for their contribution and expertise: Barbara Arroyo, Edward Chesney, Arsime Demjaha, Paolo Fusar-Poli, Fiona Gaughran, Guy Goodwin, Robert Harland, Eleanor Hinds, Juliet Hurn, Sameer Jauhar, Luke Jelen, Anne Kjerrström, John Lally, James MaCabe, Rachael McGuinness, Robert Miller, Sridhar Natesan, Toby Pillinger, Ros Ramsay, Ashvini Ramoutar, Tim Segal, Matthew Taylor and Allan Young.

COI statements

"Paul Morrison has received funding from GW pharmaceuticals in the form of unrestricted grants, speaker's fees from Otsuka, Pfizer and Valeant and consultancy fees from GW pharmaceuticals, Oxford PharmGenesis and Boehringer Ingelheim".

"David M. Taylor has received research funding and lecturing honoraria from Janssen, Otsuka, Lundbeck, Sunovion and Galen"

Philip McGuire has received research grant funding from GW Pharmaceuticals.

Psychosis

1.1 What is psychosis?

Psychiatry has always struggled with terms and definitions. Canvass the opinions of a modern community multidisciplinary team, and there are likely to be a range of opinions on what psychosis actually is [1]. Yet very few will object to the phenomenological perspective, which captures the seriousness of just what is at stake in psychosis. That is because psychosis impacts upon the highest and most personal faculties of the human mind.

In short, psychosis describes a disturbance of perception, thinking, beliefs, or selfhood in which the patient experiences a fundamental transformation in their experience of lived reality. This transformation can be terrifying as in paranoid psychoses or thrilling as in mania. Psychosis can emerge and dissipate quickly or become ingrained in the mind/brain over many months. Some patients seek safety by withdrawing from the world, whereas others attract attention to their mental state through excited, agitated, bizarre, or catatonic behaviour.

1.2 Lack of insight

The most common feature of psychosis is not hallucinations, delusions, thought disorder, paranoia or suspiciousness as is commonly believed but lack of insight [2]. Lack of insight denotes the blind-spot a patient has in regard to the falseness of their new reality and the abnormal nature of their mental state [3]. For some the term 'lack of insight' exemplifies the power imbalance within psychiatry.

Regardless of terminology, the blind-spot is what makes the care of many patients suffering psychosis particularly challenging. Why would anyone take treatment, let alone engage with mental health professionals if they think their experiences are real rather than a manifestation of psychiatric illness.

Advanced Prescribing in Psychosis, First Edition. Paul Morrison, David M. Taylor and Phillip McGuire.
© 2020 John Wiley & Sons Ltd. Published 2020 by John Wiley & Sons Ltd.

1.3   Causes of psychosis

Mental states have material correlates. For some patients, a material dysfunction is the direct cause of their psychosis. The list of causes includes endocrine disorders (e.g. *thyroid disease*), metabolic disorders (e.g. *porphyria*), auto-immune conditions (e.g. *N*-methyl-D-*aspartate*, NMDA-*receptor encephalitis*), infections (e.g. *herpes-simplex encephalitis*), epilepsy (e.g. *temporal lobe epilepsy*), nutritional deficits (e.g. *vitamin B12 deficiency*), basal ganglia disorders (e.g. *Wilson's disease*), medications (e.g. *acyclovir)*, dementias (e.g. *Alzheimer's disease*), and most common of all, psychoactive drugs, as causes [4].

The following psychoactive drugs can elicit an acute psychotic episode after a single administration: serotonin $5HT_{2A}$ receptor agonists (e.g. *lysergic acid diethylamide, LSD*), glutamate NMDA channel blockers (e.g. *ketamine),* and cannabinoid CB_1 receptor agonists (e.g. *delta-9-tetrahydrocannabinol, THC*) [5].
Repeated, heavy use of stimulants can elicit a classic paranoid psychosis by impacting upon dopamine signalling (e.g. *methamphetamine*) [5, 6].

Psychosis can occur in the following syndromes: schizophrenia, delusional disorder, bipolar disorder, post-partum psychosis, schizoaffective disorder, and depression. Psychotic experiences can also manifest in severe obsessive compulsive disorder (OCD). There are also brief, acute, full-blown psychotic episodes occurring outwith any of these syndromes, which even in the era before antipsychotic drugs, tended to show a full recovery of insight and restoration of the former reality [7, 8].
Auditory *pseudo*-hallucinations and 'paranoia' can occur in people prone to emotional instability, but insight is maintained, and the prominence of deliberate self-harm in the context of early abuse steers the formulation away from a psychotic disorder [9–11]. Indeed, psychotic-like phenomena including voices and paranoia occur in the general population, but such experiences do not overwhelm the self to the extent that there is a fundamental transformation of lived reality, and should not be over-psychologised as markers of mental illness [12–14].

Robin Murray and Jim van Os have made the elegant observation that, 'the boundaries between normal mentation, common mental disorder and schizophrenia become blurred, if positive psychotic symptoms are used as a distinguisher' [15].

Precise diagnosis might not be possible, but in some cases it is vital. For instance, psychosis arising from antibodies targeting the NMDA-receptor requires urgent immunological treatment [16]. In such cases antipsychotics and psychological therapy are of no value and lead to delays.
Given the multitude of causes of psychosis, patients require a skilled assessment and careful biopsychosocial formulation before treatment, whether pharmacological or psychological, is embarked upon [17].

1.4   Schizophrenia: loss of personality and psychosocial decline

Psychosis and schizophrenia are not synonymous. Only about one in eight patients who experience an acute psychosis will go on to develop schizophrenia over a period of three to five years [18].

Schizophrenia is not a single syndrome [19]. From the outset, the term subsumed a collection of phenotypes [20–22].

Paranoid form, dominated by psychotic symptoms.
Hebephrenic form, dominated by severe thought disorder and bizarre affect.
Catatonic form, dominated by psychomotor signs.
Simple form, dominated by severe psychosocial decline but no psychotic symptoms.

The precise definition and demarcation of schizophrenia is as uncertain as ever, and some authorities have suggested dropping the term altogether because of the associated stigma [23, 24].

On the other hand, there are a proportion of patients who exhibit such marked social decline and loss of personality for whom no alternative descriptor is forthcoming.

Many consider that psychosocial decline and loss of personality are the hallmarks of schizophrenia [25]. Essentially the same meaning is conveyed by the term, *negative symptoms*, originally formulated in nineteenth-century neurology to describe the loss of a function which is normally present in health. In schizophrenia the loss encompasses; drive, motivation, ambition, emotion, conversation, interests, family life, friendships, romantic relationships, and intellectual life [26–28].

A proportion of patients present with negative symptoms from the outset. Indeed, the drift towards psychosocial withdrawal and personality decline can precede a psychotic episode by several years [25].

Negative symptoms carry much more prognostic and diagnostic weight than the positive symptoms. Negative symptoms are commensurate with poorer long-term outcomes [29].

Schizophrenic patients with prominent negative symptoms are amongst the most psychosocially disabled, but sometimes the absence of risk alerts means that they can often be overlooked [30, 31]. Indeed, the absence or relative paucity of 'voices' and 'paranoia' in the overall clinical picture can even lead inexperienced workers to judge that there is no evidence of a mental disorder.

A relatively common error is the misdiagnosis of an autistic disorder. The negative syndrome of schizophrenia and autistic disorders are characterised by impaired social interaction. A key distinguishing feature is that autism is manifest before the age of three years, whereas a schizophrenic decline emerges in adolescence/early adulthood.

One concern, which has arisen, is that there may be a tendency towards under-recognition and under-treatment of severe and enduring mental illness, such as negative syndrome schizophrenia, and over-responding to relatively mild psychological problems [32].

1.5 Bipolar disorder

Bipolar disorder is a lifelong, episodic illness with high heritability [33] Bipolar I is defined by mania. In mania, there is an absence of insight, the cardinal feature of psychosis [33].

Bipolar patients typically recover insight between manic episodes, in that they can take a rationale perspective on their previous mental state and judge correctly that their experience of lived-reality at the time of crisis was pathological [34, 35].

Bipolar I is diagnosed after one episode of mania. Mania is characterised by a discrete period of at least one week of: persistently elevated or irritable mood; increased self-esteem or grandiosity; decreased need for sleep; more talkativeness than usual or pressure to keep talking; flight of ideas or subjective experience of racing thoughts; distractibility; increased goal-directed activity, or excessive involvement in pleasurable activities with high potential for painful results.

Bipolar II is diagnosed after one episode of hypomania + one episode of depression. Hypomania ('mini-mania') is recognised as mania which is not severe enough to cause a marked impairment in psychosocial functioning, psychosis, or to require hospitalisation. Periods of hypomania lasting one to four days are more common than prolonged episodes [36].

In the *Diagnostic and Statistical Manual of Mental Disorders* (DSM5), the presence of increased activity is a requirement for mania/hypomania. Increased activity can differentiate mania/hypomania from other illnesses [37].

1.6 Cannabis, synthetic cannabinoids, and psychosis

Clinicians who treat psychosis will be familiar with the range of patients who present with problems arising from cannabis use [38]. At least one-quarter of all new cases of psychotic illness in South London are attributable to high-potency 'skunk' cannabis [39].

Compared to traditional cannabis, skunk is high in the pro-psychotic molecule THC, but contains negligible amounts of another molecule called cannabidiol (CBD). The balance is important as CBD inhibits the psychotic effect of THC [40]. CBD also appears to have therapeutic effects in schizophrenia [41].

Acute cannabinoid psychoses are typically paranoid or manic in flavour. Less commonly, there can be hebephrenic features or motor signs such as posturing and bizarre gestures [42].

Some patients go through an acute psychosis as a result of high potency cannabinoids, but return to their lives, chastened by the intensity of their experience. Others abstain for a period, but dabble again, going through a relapse. A significant proportion of patients simply refuse to accept that cannabis has a negative impact on their mental health, and continue using the drug on a regular basis.

Two very large studies from Scandinavia found that about 50% of patients who present to emergency services with a cannabis elicited psychosis will go onto become long-term psychiatric patients [43, 44].

THC, is a partial agonist at the CB_1 receptor. The synthetic cannabinoids ('spice') are full agonists at the CB_1 receptor and have much stronger effects on the psyche, eliciting intense, florid psychoses [45]. Synthetic cannabinoids can also have a pronounced effect on heart rate and blood pressure.

An emerging concern is that the synthetic cannabinoids may be so powerful as to overwhelm the stabilising properties of antipsychotic medication.

The synthetic cannabinoids are not detected in standard drug screens, and over 150 molecules are available. Markers of synthetic cannabinoids use include confusion, slurred speech, excessive sweating, tachycardia and hypertension [46].

Complications of synthetic cannabis use include renal failure, pulmonary damage, myocardial infarction, seizures, and stroke [46].

Synthetic cannabinoids have emerged as a major problem in UK prisons [47].

Around one in seven cannabis users in the population meet criteria for dependence. High-potency cannabinoid preparations appear to have more propensity for addiction. There is a cannabis withdrawal syndrome, which resembles nicotine withdrawal. Cravings and psychomotor agitation peak at days 3–4 and diminish over 14 days [48].

Many patients who are able to sustain abstinence can make a significant recovery. The challenge, of course, is in persuading patients that the downside of their drug use far outweighs any residual upside.

In many US states and in Canada, cannabis has been legalised for recreational or medical use. Products that are high in THC with negligible CBD concentrations can be readily purchased. There are worries that cannabis-related psychiatric problems could increase in North America with the change in legislation [49].

Chapter 2

Towards evidence based treatments for psychosis

2.1 Traditional medicine

The first genuinely effective treatment for psychosis was the Indian snakeroot plant (*Rauwolfia serpentina*) which contains reserpine. The plant was used in the Ayurvedic system of India and traditional Chinese medicine. Clinical trials were conducted in the West in the 1950s and showed that reserpine was effective in schizophrenia [50].

2.2 The randomised controlled trial

The randomised controlled trial (RCT) is the only guaranteed way to establish whether a treatment actually works or not. A well-performed RCT eliminates bias, the natural tendency to assume that one's intervention is effective.

Many of the first proper clinical trials in medicine were in the field of psychiatry. The benefits of lithium for mania and chlorpromazine for schizophrenia were confirmed in RCTs by 1954 [51, 52]. Perhaps more importantly, trials also revealed where existing practice was of no benefit. Case in point is insulin coma therapy which was assumed to work, came with elaborate guidelines, and was widely rolled-out to the extent that whole wards in the UK were adapted to accommodate six treatments per week for up to two months. When subjected to the demands of the scientific method however, insulin coma therapy was shown to be of no value and was rapidly discontinued [53].

The lesson of insulin coma therapy is that if an intervention fails to outperform a placebo control in a large sample, there is little value for patients in commissioning such treatment.

Advanced Prescribing in Psychosis, First Edition. Paul Morrison, David M. Taylor and Phillip McGuire.
© 2020 John Wiley & Sons Ltd. Published 2020 by John Wiley & Sons Ltd.

2.3   The roots of community care

The emergence of genuinely effective treatments such as lithium and chlorpromazine ushered in a radical change in service delivery. In the first years of the NHS, 40% of hospital beds were for the mentally ill. The introduction of antipsychotic drugs led to a massive reduction in the number of patients who needed to be in psychiatric hospital [54, 55]. Pharmacological treatments for major psychiatric disorders were so powerful as to effect enormous social change, but this fact has tended to be overlooked with the passage of time [56].

It is readily apparent that many patients need more than pharmaceuticals and that a package of psychosocial rehabilitation is needed to recover any quality of life [57]. This is especially clear for schizophrenic patients disabled by negative symptoms and poverty. A concern is that there is under-allocation of resource for those with a severe and enduring mental illness, in parallel with over-treatment of relatively mild psychological problems [32].

2.4   Treatment algorithms versus personalised care

Modern trials in psychiatry often compare whether one pharmaceutical outperforms another. On this basis, there has been an effort to rank the wide range of different antipsychotic compounds currently available for the treatment of psychosis [58]. Clinical judgement draws not just on rankings of drugs from population data, but also on the specific characteristics and particular circumstances of the individual patient. The task of the prescriber is to integrate population data and patient-specific factors.

The antipsychotics

3.1 General principles in the pharmacology of psychosis

All of the antipsychotic drugs which are in use for patients have a wide safety window and proven efficacy in large controlled trials. Table 3.1 lists the general principles in the pharmacology of psychosis. They all block the dopamine type-2 receptor (D_2) receptor which underlies their antipsychotic effect [59].

Reserpine, a naturally occurring molecule and the first antipsychotic is an exception. Reserpine works in a slightly different way, by depleting nerve varicosities of monoamine neurotransmitters, dopamine included, but by the end of the 1950s there was a consensus that the D_2 receptor blockers were more effective in schizophrenia, and the use of reserpine diminished [60].

The D_2 receptor blockers differ from each other in their propensity to act as additional receptors, producing effects which may be desirable or unwanted [61]. Sedation, for example, may be welcome in the agitated setting of an acute psychosis, but be unwanted once the psychosis has resolved (Table 3.2).

When selecting an antipsychotic drug, it is worth distinguishing between the treatment of a psychotic episode and maintenance treatment. In an acute psychotic episode, the emphasis is on prompt relief of symptoms. In the maintenance stage, the emphasis is on avoiding side-effects so that a patient is more likely to adhere to treatment and be at lower risk of relapse [62–64]. Non-adherence to medication is the largest predictor of relapse [65].

Personalised medicine necessarily involves trial and error, with feedback and adjustment. Psycho-education is vital. Ideally the process should tend towards the patient being equipped to make their own pharmaceutical choices. Sharing research evidence in an intuitive format, and a collaborative approach to decision-making can enhance the therapeutic relationship [66].

Several antipsychotic drugs have antidepressant, anxiolytic and anti-obsessional properties, which the over-arching term '*antipsychotic*' fails to capture [67–69]. Moves

Advanced Prescribing in Psychosis, First Edition. Paul Morrison, David M. Taylor and Phillip McGuire.
© 2020 John Wiley & Sons Ltd. Published 2020 by John Wiley & Sons Ltd.

Table 3.1 General principles in the pharmacology of psychosis.

1. Clarify the clinical picture
History, examination, collateral history, investigation, formulation & diagnosis if possible.
Organic cause v functional? Acute v insidious onset? Family history? Drug misuse? Schizophrenia-like? Manic? Schizoaffective? Psychotic depression? Borderline? Risk to self/others?

2. Be clear about the goals of treatment at different stages:
An acute psychotic episode: Prompt, safe, symptom control.
Maintenance stage, minimise the risk of side-effects.

3. First episode psychosis?
Baseline assessments, including urine drug screen (UDS).
Be mindful that first-episode patients can be sensitive to antipsychotics – 'Low and slow'.
Carefully review the response to a particular dose of medicine and tailor for the individual.

4. The presence of acute agitation?
Select a sedative antipsychotic which blocks histamine H1 receptors?
Combine an antipsychotic with a short course of a benzodiazepine?[a] Table 3.4.
Combine an antipsychotic with a short course of Z-drug for insomnia? Table 3.4

5. Relapse?
Carry out appropriate assessments. e.g. Plasma drug level monitoring. UDS.
Review the notes. Which treatments and doses were effective and well-tolerated in previous episodes?

6. Psycho-education is vital for the therapeutic relationship:
Highlight immediate benefits of treatment, e.g. 'better sleep, less anxiety'.
Discuss evolving benefits, e.g. 'better focus, less paranoia, able to get on with life again'.
Alert patients in advance about the most common side effects and discuss a contingency plan.
Ideally, patients will be empowered to choose their own pharmaceutical treatment.

7. Maintenance treatment:
Non-adherence is predicted by the failure of insight to recover.
Non-adherence to medication is the strongest predictor of relapse.
Depot formulations are superior to tablets in reducing the chances of relapse.
Adherence therapy is effective, and reduces relapse.

8. Individualised care:
Tailor treatment towards the specific needs of the individual patient.
The tapering and possible cessation of antipsychotics should be based on individual factors, rather than a one-size-fits-all approach. Discontinuation carries a high risk of relapse over the first 3 years. A high antipsychotic load may be associated with poorer long-term functional outcomes.

[a] Need >2 hours between intra-Muscular (IM) olanzapine + IM benzodiazepine due to risk of respiratory depression.

are afoot to develop a new classification system of all psychoactive drugs, based on neuroscience, which captures the nuances of each molecule and takes receptor pharmacology into account (www.nbn2.com).

3.2 Neurotransmitters and receptors

The antipsychotics bind to many members of the large super-family of G-protein coupled receptors (GPCRs) [70]. Having evolved from a common ancestor, all of the GPCRs share structural features [71]. Some of the antipsychotics are very promiscuous and bind to a multitude of receptors, others are far more selective for the dopamine D_2 receptor.

For clinical purposes, the effects of an individual antipsychotic can be predicted from the receptor binding profile. Often, there is a direct mapping between a receptor and a

Table 3.2 Comparative receptor affinity of commonly prescribed antipsychotics.

Antipsychotic drug	Dopamine D2 receptor affinity *antipsychotic effect motor side effects*	Histamine H1 receptor affinity	Noradrenergic α1 receptor affinity *postural hypotension ? utility against nightmares in PTSD*	Muscarinic (M1–M5) receptor affinity *dry mouth blurred vision constipation urinary retention anti-parkinsonian*
Aripiprazole	++++ (partial agonist)	+	+	0
Brexpiprazole	++++ (partial agonist)	++	+++	+
Cariprazine	++++ (partial agonist)	++	+	0
Flupentixol	++++	++++	+++	+
Trifluoperazine	++++	+	++	+
Zuclopenthixol	++++	+	+++	0
Amisulpride	+++	0	0	0
Chlorpromazine	+++	++++	++++	++
Haloperidol	+++	0	++	0
Lurasidone	+++	0	++	0
Risperidone	+++	+++	+++	0
Asenapine	+++	+++	+++	0
Ziprasidone	+++	++	++	0
Iloperidone	+++	+	++++	0
Olanzapine	++	+++	+	++ but rarely causes anticholinergic effects in trials/practice
Clozapine	+	+++	+++	++ partial agonist: hyper-salivation & urinary incontinence
Quetiapine	+	+++	+++	++ (*norquetiapine*)

Affinity: ++++ Very High (< 1 nm); +++ High (1–10 nM); ++ Moderate (10–100 nM); + Low (100–1000 nM); 0 non-significant (>1000 nM).
Source: Ref: PDSP database (University of North Carolina, USA)

particular effect. This can be particularly useful when a new antipsychotic emerges, before clinical experience with the new molecule has accrued.

Well characterised mappings:
Dopamine D_2 antagonist – antipsychotic.
Noradrenaline $α_1$ antagonist – hypotension.
Histamine H_1 antagonist – sedation.

Acetylcholine M_1–M_5 antagonist – anti-parkinsonian.
Serotonin $5HT_{1A}$ partial agonist – anxiolytic.
hERG potassium channel blockade – long QT_C.

Hypothesised mappings:
Serotonin 5HT2C antagonist – weight gain.
Acetylcholine M3 antagonist – type II diabetes.
Serotonin 5HT7 antagonist – antidepressant.
Serotonin 5HT2A antagonist – antipsychotic.
Acetylcholine M4 agonist – antipsychotic.

Some antipsychotics have a higher preference for other receptors over dopamine D_2 (Table 3.2). Quetiapine, for example, prefers histamine H_1 over D_2 to the extent that the H_1 receptor population will be saturated by doses of quetiapine which have a negligible impact upon the D_2 receptor pool [72]. Clinically, this means that sedation is inevitable if quetiapine is used as an antipsychotic, at least in the early weeks of treatment before the brain adapts.

Clozapine in particular has a preference for numerous G-protein coupled receptors ahead of D_2, including the serotonin $5HT_{2c}$ and acetylcholine M_3 receptors (Psychoactive Drug Screening Program (PDSP) database, University of North Carolina, USA). Binding to $5HT_{2c}$ and M_3 is unavoidable at doses of clozapine needed for an antipsychotic effect.
See Table 3.7 for the receptor binding profile of the most commonly prescribed antipsychotics, ranked according to affinity.

There was hope that molecules targeting the glutamate system would become a new class of antipsychotic medication. It was even anticipated that glutamate drugs would be effective for the negative and cognitive symptoms of schizophrenia. Despite early promises however, large trials of glutamate drugs (*(i) mGluR2/3 agonists and (ii) GlyT1 inhibitors*) failed to show any therapeutic benefits for schizophrenia [73, 74].

3.3 Choosing drugs

It is only partially true that drugs can be ranked according to their efficacy in schizophrenia. In the treatment-resistant state, clozapine is superior to all other antipsychotics [75]. Otherwise, there is little difference between antipsychotic drugs in terms of efficacy [76–78]. Some authorities and trials place olanzapine slightly ahead of the rest of the pack in terms of efficacy [79, 80], and there is some evidence that 'higher doses' of olanzapine (25–$45\,mg\,d^{-1}$) may even be as effective as clozapine in the treatment-resistant state [81].

For schizophrenia, the first generation (typical) drugs are equally as effective as the second generation (atypical) class. The notion of typical and atypical classes which emerged in the 1990s should become redundant, having little basis in molecular or clinical pharmacology [82].

It was previously suggested that:

a. Parkinsonism was unlikely with atypical antipsychotics because atypicals have an ability to block serotonin $5HT_{2A}$ receptors [83].

However, some atypicals (such as risperidone) can induce Parkinsonism, while the prototypical typical antipsychotic chlorpromazine blocks $5HT_{2A}$ receptors. Parkinsonism appears to be more a function of antipsychotic dose and hence the degree of D_2 rather than $5HT_{2A}$ receptor binding.

b. Atypicals were unlikely to induce high serum prolactin levels.

However, some atypicals such as risperidone and amisulpride can cause high prolactin levels [84].

c. Typicals cause motor side effects whereas atypicals lead to weight gain.

However, chlorpromazine (typical class) can cause weight gain, while aripiprazole and lurasidone (atypical class) tend to be relatively weight neutral [85, 86].

It thus makes more sense to examine each antipsychotic drug in its own right and abandon the typical/atypical distinction [87, 82]. Ideally, the choice of antipsychotic drug should be tailored towards the needs of each patient at a particular time [82, 88–90].

- Table 3.3 Antipsychotics for an acute episode.
- Table 3.4 Adjunctive medication for an acute episode.
- Table 3.5 Rapid tranquillisation
- Table 3.6 Clopixol acuphase (zuclopenthixol acetate)
- Table 3.7 Antipsychotics for the maintenance phase.
- Appendix 1. The pharmacokinetics of selected psychotropics.
- Appendix 3. Physical health monitoring for patients prescribed antipsychotics
- Appendix 4. Physical health monitoring for patients prescribed mood stabilisers.

3.4   Acute psychotic episodes

The properties of antipsychotic drugs that are commonly used to treat an acute psychotic episode are shown in Table 3.3.

Prescribing for acute psychotic episodes takes place within the context of a comprehensive history, investigation, and an appraisal of any previous treatment. Given the ubiquity of drug misuse, and the ability of illicit drugs to elicit a psychosis, efforts should always be made to obtain a urine drug screen (UDS) for illicit substances.

For patients presenting with psychosis for the first time, an antipsychotic free assessment period is desirable. An antipsychotic free period offers time for clarification of the clinical picture and where possible, a diagnosis (Section 1.3). Distress may supervene, although this can often be relieved with a benzodiazepine or a sedative antihistamine alone, rather than proceeding to antipsychotics straight away.

When a patient's clinical records show that an antipsychotic was prescribed in an acute setting, this can be taken as supporting a diagnosis of a major psychotic syndrome. However, it may be that the immediate relief of distress or agitation was the impetus for prescribing.

Table 3.3 Antipsychotics for an acute psychotic episode.

Drug (oral preparations) Dose range	Properties
Amisulpride 50–1200 mg d^{-1}	Non-sedating.
Aripiprazole 5–30 mg d^{-1}	Non-sedating. Dose-related akathisia
Cariprazine 1.5–6 mg d^{-1}	Dose-related akathisia
Brexpiprazole 0.5–4 mg d^{-1}	Less akathisia than other D$_2$ partial agonists.
Quetiapine 50–750 mg d^{-1} (in mania max. is 800 mg d^{-1})	Potent sedative. Weak antipsychotic until higher doses reached. Requires titration to avoid postural hypotension. ■ Propensity for rapid weight gain over a period of weeks.
Trifluoperazine 4–20 mg d^{-1} (max 30 mg d^{-1})	■ Dose-related motor side effects.
Risperidone 1–16 mg d^{-1}	Requires titration to avoid postural hypotension. Oro-dispersible formulation available ■ Dose-related motor side effects.
Ziprasidone 20–80 mg bd.	■ ↑ QTc by >20 ms Non-sedating. ■ Dose-related motor side effects.
Iloperidone 1 mg bd, increments of 2 mg d^{-1} to 6–12 mg bd.	Requires titration to avoid postural hypotension.
Haloperidol 1.5–20 mg d^{-1} *No evidence of any benefit >6 mg d^{-1}*	■ Dose-related motor side effects. Requirement for prior ECG
Chlorpromazine 75–1000 mg d^{-1}	Potent sedative. ■ Dose-related motor side effects. ■ Propensity for rapid weight gain over a period of weeks.
Flupentixol 3–18 mg d^{-1}	■ Dose-related motor side effects. Avoid in agitated or excitable patients, may exacerbate these features.
Olanzapine 5–20 mg d^{-1}	Potent sedative. Better efficacy than the others (clozapine and treatment resistance aside). Negligible risk of motor side effects. Oro-dispersible formulation available. ■ Propensity for rapid weight gain over a period of weeks.

Titrate doses versus efficacy and tolerability on a case-by-case basis.
If no improvements at 2–3 weeks: – Review dose. Exclude drug interactions. Check adherence. Plasma level monitoring.
Revisit the history. Exclude organic cause. Urine drug screen.
Consider switch of antipsychotic.
If failure to respond to adequate trials of two antipsychotics.
Consider clozapine
Source: Data from electronic medicines compendium (EMC). www.medicines.org.uk/emc.

On the other hand, there is little rationale for delaying antipsychotic treatment if the clinical picture indicates a paranoid psychotic illness emerging from a clear-cut pro-dromal period. Delaying antipsychotic treatment (*albeit over a timescale of months, rather than days*) can result in poorer long-term outcomes in terms of symptoms and functioning [91–93].

All of the antipsychotic drugs are effective in an acute psychosis. The relief of distress and agitation often takes priority.

3.4.1   Olanzapine in acute psychotic episodes

Olanzapine has properties which make it a popular choice for acute psychotic episodes. It is sedative and a potent antipsychotic. But perhaps the most desirable property of olanzapine in an acute setting (*where higher doses of antipsychotic may be needed*) is that it has a negligible risk of motor reactions [94, 95].

The majority of clinicians recognise that, for most patients, olanzapine is not an ideal product beyond the acute stage. Many patients start to show rapid weight gain in the initial weeks of treatment [96, 97], although add-on metformin [98], Glucagon-like peptide-1 receptor agonists [99] or low-dose aripiprazole may mitigate weight-gain [100] (see Section 6.1).

In the aftermath of an acute episode, there is a case for transferring a patient away from olanzapine to a relatively weight neutral antipsychotic. Cross-tapering is preferable, typically over a period of four to six weeks. The key points are that individualised care is needed rather than a one-size fits all approach and that follow-up appointments should be frequent during the cross-over to allow fine-tuning.

Note that the withdrawal of olanzapine can precipitate transient, but marked insomnia, as the sleep centres re-adjust to the absence of olanzapine and its replacement by a non-sedative or activating antipsychotic, such as aripiprazole. A short course of a Z-drug (Table 3.4) can facilitate the cross-over.

Some prescribers may have an eye towards the longer term from the outset, selecting an antipsychotic that has less propensity for weight gain, and managing acute insomnia and agitation with adjunctive medication (Table 3.4).

3.4.2   Antipsychotic dosing in acute psychotic episodes

Antipsychotic doses should be tailored for each individual patient.[88, 82] Efficacy and tolerability should be assessed after initiation of a drug or following a change of dose.

In regard to dosing, the recommended approach is to titrate up and observe, rather than to overmedicate and taper down, given that there is considerable variation in how individual patients respond to a given dose of drug. A one size fits all approach to dose selection will inevitably result in a proportion of patients experiencing dystonia, akathisia and Parkinsonism, which can taint the initial experience of mental health care [82].

Table 3.4 Adjunctive medication for an acute psychotic episode.

Drug	Pharmacokinetics	Properties
Z-drug class		
Zolpidem oral 5–10 mg nocte	T_{max}: 0.5–3 h Half-life 2–3 h CYP3A4	Sedative hypnotic Not anxiolytic
Zopiclone oral 3.75–7.5 mg nocte	Tmax: 1.5–2 h Half-life 3.5–6.5 h CYP3A4 and CYP2C8	
Sedative H$_1$ antihistamine		
Promethazine oral 25–100 mg Licence: 25–50 mg (as antiemetic) Usual doses: 25–100 mg	Tmax: 2–3 h Half-life 12–19 h	Sedative hypnotic Not anxiolytic D$_2$ antagonist effect. Anti-muscarinic effects. - No sense in adding to high H$_1$ affinity antipsychotics (Table 3.2).
Benzodiazepine class		
Lorazepam oral 1–4 mg d^{-1}	Tmax: 2 h Half-life: 12 h glucuronidation	Sedative hypnotic Anxiolytic Avoid prolonged use (>2–3 wk) ▪ Clonazepam and diazepam can accumulate.
Clonazepam oral 0.5–2 mg d^{-1} Licence: up to 8 mg d^{-1} (in epilepsy)	Tmax: 1–4 h Half-life: 20–60 h Mean 30 h CYP2C19	
Diazepam oral 5–20 mg d^{-1} Licence: up to 30 mg d^{-1} in anxiety	Tmax: 0.5–1.5 h Half-life: 20–100 h Active metabolites CYP2C19 and CYP3A4	
Midazolam buccal 10 mg	Tmax: 0.5 h Half-life: 1.5–2.5 h CYP3A4	

Source: Data from electronic medicines compendium (EMC). www.medicines.org.uk/emc.

Older adults who developed a schizophrenia-like psychosis later in life (over 60) have been shown to make significant improvements when treated with low dose amisulpride (100 mg d^{-1}) [101].

The ward and the home treatment team (HTT) are ideal settings for the titration and ongoing close assessment of drug effects as a function of dose. Frequent review is key.

Knowledge of the pharmacokinetic properties of a drug can inform prescribing. In general, the plasma level of a drug accumulates with repeated doses, reaching a relatively steady plateau by the time of approximately five half-lives (Appendix 1).

3.4.3 Timescale of response in acute psychotic episodes

It used to be believed that the antipsychotics take several weeks to work in paranoid psychoses. However, benefits are typically seen within the first 24–48 hours and throughout the first week.

By the second week there should be signs of at least minimal improvement [102]. If there are no improvements [103]:

Review the dose. Exclude drug interactions.
Check adherence. Plasma level monitoring.
Revisit the history. Exclude organic cause. UDS.
Consider a switch of antipsychotic.
If failure to respond to adequate trials of two antipsychotics.
Consider clozapine.

3.4.4 Very agitated patients

Sometimes patients are so overwhelmed and agitated by psychosis that they begin to act upon their experiences. Events can escalate quickly. Understandably, aggression can be employed as a defence, carrying a risk of physical harm to self and others. The Maudsley protocol for rapid tranquilisation is detailed in Table 3.5.

Clopixol acuphase can be helpful for patients whose agitation has required repeated short-acting IM injections. Acuphase has favourable pharmacokinetic properties in such circumstances. The desired effects of tranquilisation and sedation last days rather than hours. The protocol for acuphase treatment is detailed in Table 3.6.

Table 3.5 Rapid tranquillisation.

Maudsley Protocol: [104]
De-escalation, time-out, secure placement if appropriate.
Offer oral meds:
    lorazepam 1–2 mg
    repeat after 45–60 min
    Buccal midazolam 10 mg
    oral antipsychotic if not already taking a regular antipsychotic
        olanzapine 10 mg
        haloperidol 5 mg (ECG recommended)
Consider IM meds:
    lorazepam 1–2 mg
    have flumazenil close to hand for respiratory depression
    promethazine 50 mg
    olanzapine 10 mg
    need >2 h between IM olanzapine and IM benzodiazepine
    aripiprazole 9.75 mg
    haloperidol 5 mg (ECG recommended)
    need IM procyclidine close to hand for dystonia
    haloperidol should be the last drug considered
    combine with IM lorazepam or IM promethazine
Seek expert advice.

Table 3.6 Clopixol acuphase (zuclopenthixol acetate).

Used for the short-term management of acute psychoses in patients who have had repeated injections of IM olanzapine or IM haloperidol.
Avoid in: neuroleptic naive patients, pregnancy, hepatic or renal impairment, cardiac disease, CNS depression.
Dose: 50–150 mg then 50–150 mg after 2–3 days if needed.
Maximum cumulative dose 400 mg. Maximum duration 2 weeks. Maximum injections 4
Pharmacokinetics: T_{max} 36 h; At three days post-injection levels are 1/3 of C_{max}.
Typically, sedation begins two hours after injection. Effects last up to 72 h.

Source: Data from electronic medicines compendium (EMC). www.medicines.org.uk/emc.

3.5   The maintenance phase: relapse prevention

The properties of commonly used antipsychotics, in the context of the maintenance phase are shown in Table 3.7.

The primary aim of treatment in the maintenance phase is relapse prevention. Lack of insight predicts non-adherence to medication [105–109]. Rates of non-adherence are approximately 50% [110].

Non-adherence to medication is the main factor leading to a relapse of psychosis [65, 111–114]. One study found that in the first year of recovery, relapse rates were: off medication 77% versus on-medication 3% [115]. Another study showed that patients who discontinue medication have a fivefold higher chance of relapse compared to those who continue medication [113].

Other predictors of relapse are the presence of substance abuse, critical comments and poor pre-morbid adjustment [114, 107].
Even temporary periods of non-adherence (not just complete discontinuation) appear to significantly increase the risk of relapse [116].

Each relapse can be traumatic in itself. For many patients repeated relapse means progressive social and functional decline. Moreover, the pathology of perception, thinking, beliefs and selfhood which constitutes psychosis can become stubbornly ingrained and less responsive to treatment [117, 118].

Even in the absence of side effects, taking a drug every day for months or years is challenging. Care should be taken to reduce side effects to an absolute minimum [64]. The ideal antipsychotic drug for the maintenance phase is the medication that is most acceptable to the individual patient [119, 82, 120].

In comparison to treatment as usual, adherence therapy, given in individual or group settings can improve adherence, improve symptoms, improve functioning, improve quality of life, and reduce the rate of re-admission to hospital [121–126]. Adherence therapy also appears to reduce overall healthcare costs [127, 128].

3.5.1   Beyond the early years: more harm than good?

There are clear benefits of maintenance antipsychotic medication in the early years of a first episode psychosis, but there has been a worry that, after the first years, antipsychotics may do more harm than good [112]. Robust long-term studies are needed to

Table 3.7 Antipsychotics for the maintenance phase.

Drug Dose range	Receptor profile in order of affinity	Upside	Downside
Amisulpride Licence: 50–1200 mg d^{-1} Positive symptoms: 400–1200 mg d^{-1} Negative symptoms: 50–300 mg d^{-1}	D_2 antagonist $5HT_7$ antagonist	Weight gain 0/+. Non-sedative. ? Efficacy for negative symptoms. Antidepressant properties *at low doses*.	High prolactin. EPSEs
Aripiprazole 5–30 mg d^{-1}	D_2 partial agonist $5HT_{2A}$ antagonist $5HT_{1A}$ partial agonist $5HT_7$ antagonist $5HT_{2C}$ partial agonist α_2 antagonist	Weight gain 0/+. Non-sedative. Can normalise high prolactin. Low propensity for sexual side effects. Available as long-acting depot. Antidepressant properties	Akathisia. Nausea. Insomnia.
Quetiapine Starting dose: 50 mg 150–750 mg d^{-1} *Norquetiapine (metabolite of quetiapine)*	H_1 antagonist α_1 antagonist D_2 antagonist at higher doses $5HT_{2C}$ antagonist *NET inhibitor* M_1 *antagonist*	Low risk of Parkinsonian side effects. Effective in bipolar depression. Useful for borderline states. Low propensity for sexual side effects.	Sedation. Weight gain++ Dyslipidemia. Hyperglycemia. Postural hypotension.
Olanzapine Licence: 5–20 mg d^{-1} First episode: 5–20 mg d^{-1} Multi-episode: 7.5–20 mg d^{-1}	H_1 antagonist $5HT_{2A}$ antagonist $5HT_{2C}$ inverse agonist D_2 antagonist M_1–M_5 antagonist	Absence of Parkinsonian side effects. ? Better efficacy than others, (clozapine and treatment resistance aside).	Sedation. ! Weight gain+++ Dyslipidemia. Hyperglycemia. Risk of type II diabetes. (Depot preparation available, but problematic to use in routine practice).
Risperidone Starting dose: 2 mg Licence: 2–16 mg d^{-1} First episode: 1–3 mg d^{-1} Multi-episode: 3–6 mg d^{-1}	$5HT_{2A}$ inverse agonist D_2 antagonist $5HT_7$ antagonist α_1 antagonist $5HT_{2C}$ inverse agonist H_1 antagonist α_2 antagonist	Usually well-tolerated *at low dose*. Available as long-acting depot.	EPSEs Risk of tardive dyskinesia. High prolactin. Weight gain+ Erectile dysfunction. Postural hypotension.
Chlorpromazine Licence: 75–1000 mg d^{-1} First episode: 200 mg d^{-1} Multi-episode: 300 mg d^{-1}	H_1 antagonist α_1 antagonist D_2 antagonist $5HT_{2A}$ antagonist $5HT_{2C}$ antagonist M_1–M_5 antagonist		EPSEs Risk of tardive dyskinesia. High prolactin. Sedation. Weight gain++ Hyperglycemia. Dry mouth, constipation. Postural hypotension. Photosensitivity.

CHAPTER 3

(Continued)

Table 3.7 (Continued)

Drug Dose range	Receptor profile in order of affinity	Upside	Downside
Trifluoperazine Range: 4–20 mg d^{-1} First episode: 10 mg d^{-1} Multi-episode: 15 mg	D_2 antagonist $5HT_{2A}$ antagonist α_1 antagonist	Weight gain 0/+. Non-sedative.	EPSEs Risk of tardive dyskinesia. High prolactin. Dry mouth, constipation. Postural hypotension.
Haloperidol Range: 2–20 mg d^{-1} First episode: 2–4 mg Multi-episode: 10 mg d^{-1}	D_2 antagonist $5HT_{2A}$ antagonist α_1 antagonist	Weight gain 0/+. Non-sedative. Available as long-acting depot.	! EPSEs Risk of tardive dyskinesia. High prolactin. Agitation. Insomnia.
Lurasidone 37–148 mg d^{-1}	$5HT_7$ antagonist D_2 antagonist $5HT_{2A}$ antagonist α_2 antagonist $5HT_{1A}$ partial agonist	Weight gain 0/+. Effective in bipolar depression.	Akathisia. Sedation. Needs to be taken with/ after a meal
Clozapine starting dose: 12.5 mg maintenance: 200–450 mg d^{-1} max: 900 mg d^{-1} Guided by plasma levels. Target >0.35–0.5 mg l^{-1} (Trough).	H_1 antagonist α_1 antagonist $5HT_{2A}$ antagonist $5HT_{2C}$ inverse agonist M_1–M_5 partial agonist $5HT_7$ antagonist D_2 antagonist *at higher doses*	Efficacy in treatment-resistant cases. Efficacy for negative symptoms. Absence of Parkinsonian side-effects. Anti-suicidal effect. Effective treatment for tardive dyskinesia (TD)	Sedation. ! Weight gain+++ Dyslipidemia. Hyperglycemia. Risk of type II diabetes. Tachycardia. Hyper-salivation. Risk of neutropenia and need for blood tests. Rebound psychosis. Myocarditis. Cardiomyopathy. Constipation.
Flupentixol 3–18 mg d^{-1}	D_2 antagonist H_1 antagonist α_1 antagonist α_2 antagonist	Available as long-acting depot. Possible antidepressant properties.	EPSEs Risk of tardive Dyskinesia. High prolactin.
Brexpiprazole Adjunct in depression starting dose: 0.5–1 mg d^{-1} target dose: 2 mg d^{-1} max 3 mg d^{-1} Schizophrenia: (2–4 mg d^{-1}) starting dose: 1 mg d^{-1}, days 1–4 then 2 mg d^{-1}, days 5–7 4 mg d^{-1}, day 8	$5HT_{1A}$ partial agonist α_1 antagonist D_2 partial agonist $5HT_{2A}$ antagonist H_1 antagonist	? Efficacy for negative symptoms. Antidepressant properties. weight gain 0/+.	Akathisia, but probably less so than other D_2 partial agonists Postural hypotension.

Table 3.7 (Continued)

Drug Dose range	Receptor profile in order of affinity	Upside	Downside
Cariprazine starting dose: 1.5 mg d^{-1} 1.5–6 mg d^{-1}	D$_2$ partial agonist 5HT$_{1A}$ partial agonist 5HT$_{2A}$ antagonist H$_1$ antagonist 5HT$_{2C}$ inverse agonist at higher doses	? Efficacy for negative symptoms. Maintained efficacy with missed doses because of very long half-life of cariprazine and its active metabolite. ? Can normalise high prolactin. Weight gain 0/+. (Antidepressant properties under investigation)	Akathisia EPSEs Insomnia
Ziprasidone 20–80 mg b.d.	5HT$_{2A}$ antagonist 5HT$_{2C}$ partial agonist D$_2$ antagonist 5HT$_{1A}$ partial agonist 5HT$_7$ antagonist α$_1$ antagonist H$_1$ antagonist	Weight gain 0/+	! ↑ QTc by >20 ms Insomnia EPSEs Risk of tardive dyskinesia
Asenapine Sub-lingual 5–10 mg b.d.	5HT$_{2C}$ antagonist 5HT$_{2A}$ antagonist 5HT$_7$ antagonist H$_1$ antagonist H$_2$ antagonist α$_1$ antagonist α$_2$ antagonist D$_2$ antagonist 5HT$_{1A}$ partial agonist		Sedation EPSEs Weight gain+ Oral hypoesthesia Postural hypotension
Iloperidone Starting dose: 1 mg bd. Slow titration to minimise postural hypotension. Increments of no more than 2 mg d^{-1}. 6–12 mg bd.	α$_1$ antagonist 5HT$_{2A}$ antagonist D$_2$ antagonist 5HT$_7$ antagonist	Low risk of Parkinsonian side effects.	! Postural hypotension. Sedation Weight gain+

KEY:
D$_2$ antagonist – antipsychotic, high prolactin, motor side effects
α$_1$ antagonist – postural hypotension, efficacy against nightmares in post-traumatic stress disorder (PTSD).
α$_2$ antagonist – antidepressant, limits hypotension from α$_1$ blockade.
norepinephrine transporter (NET) inhibitor (*noradrenaline re-uptake inhibition*) – antidepressant.
H$_1$ antagonist – sedation, weight gain.
5HT$_{1A}$ partial agonist – anxiolytic.
5HT$_{2A}$ antagonist – antipsychotic activity?? anti-parkinsonian? pro-cognitive??
5HT$_{2C}$ inverse agonist/antagonist – weight gain.
5HT$_7$ antagonist – antidepressant?
M$_1$–M$_5$ partial agonist/antagonist – anti-parkinsonian, constipation, urinary retention (antagonist), urinary incontinence (partial agonist), blurred vision, dry mouth (antagonist), hyper-salivation (partial agonist), tachycardia.
Source: Data from: PDSP database (University of North Carolina, USA).Electronic medicines compendium (EMC). www.medicines.org.uk/emc.

address the issue [129] and have started to appear, but much more data is needed to guide practice in such a vital area.

In an eight-year follow-up of over 8700 patients hospitalised in Finland for first-episode schizophrenia, those who continued antipsychotics had lower relapse and lower mortality rates compared to those who discontinued antipsychotics; within one year, within one to two years, within two to five years, and after five years [130].

In a trial from Hong-Kong, patients (n = 178) whose first episode had responded fully to quetiapine were randomised to a maintenance versus a discontinuation group. At 10-year follow-up, patients in the discontinuation group had a higher risk of a having had a poor clinical outcome [131].

One quite common approach in practice is to weigh up the clinical picture in each individual and taper the antipsychotic dose to minimise side effects [64]. This strategy is supported by some recent data:

One hundred and three patients were followed up over seven years. It was found that those allocated to a treatment reduction/discontinuation arm had better functional outcomes than those maintained on the same dose of medication [132]. The maintenance group continued on an average haloperidol equivalent dose of 3.6 mg d^{-1}, the reduction/discontinuation group on an average of 2.2 mg d^{-1}. The authors suggested that a lower antipsychotic load may result in better functional capacity [132].

Some patients who have remained well and recovered insight will elect to discontinue their antipsychotic medication themselves, after discussion and reflection. A proportion will do well, but others will suffer another relapse. At present, it is not possible to differentiate between these two groups prospectively. However, a diagnosis of schizophrenia, a long duration of illness and poor premorbid functioning are associated with a greater risk of relapse [133].

Ideally, the tapering and cessation of medication should be as slow as possible. A relapse may take weeks and months to emerge. Perhaps the most important aspects are ongoing monitoring and making sure safety nets are in place should things deteriorate.

3.6   The utility of long-acting depot antipsychotics

Antipsychotics delivered in the form of a long-acting intramuscular depot have a number of advantages over orally administered formulations.

Long-acting depot achieves stable concentrations of drug in the bloodstream. For oral formulations, dosing can be highly irregular with periods of time either on-drug (*adherence monitored by home treatment team or ward*) or completely off-drug (*non-adherence*) leading to extreme fluctuations in blood concentrations [134].

In naturalistic trials, relapse rates are considerably lower with long-acting depot compared to oral formulations [135–139]. For example, in an epidemiological study of approximately 30 000 patients in Sweden, the relapse rate was 20–30% lower in patients treated with a long-acting depot antipsychotics compared to those treated with the equivalent oral formulations [140].

A recent clinical trial involving over 80 patients found that the chance of relapse over the year following a first psychotic episode was 7% for patients who were randomly allocated to depot risperidone versus 50% for patients randomised to oral risperidone [141].

Long-acting depot remains in the system for many weeks, which means that there is usually sufficient time to carefully monitor patients who discontinue or miss a dose of depot and put a plan in place to avoid a crisis. In contrast, often the first indication that a patient has discontinued their oral medication is the abrupt re-emergence of a florid psychosis, necessitating emergency admission to hospital.

Long-acting depot antipsychotics have advantages over oral treatment for avoiding relapse in psychotic disorders. However, only about one-half of patients taking oral antipsychotics will be informed about the availability of a depot, which may reflect the negative assumptions of clinical staff [142]. Negative perceptions of depots may be partly derived from previous experience with high doses of first-generation compounds.

3.7   Principles of long-acting depot antipsychotic prescribing

The pharmacokinetics of commonly used long-acting depot antipsychotics are shown in Table 3.8.

Long-acting depots are ideal for relapse prevention, but have the disadvantage of poor fine-grained control. On initiation of treatment, there can be delays of several months before steady-state levels in the bloodstream are achieved [143]. Similarly, there is a time lag after any dose adjustment until a new steady-state emerges. It can thus take four months or more to refine depot treatment for an individual patient.

The key advantage of depot over oral medication is in the longer term: reducing relapse rates, rather than the prompt relief of acute psychotic symptoms [137, 134]. It is sensible to avoid being over-zealous with the initial doses of a depot. For some drugs, oral medication can be tried first to establish tolerability. A particularly depressing scenario is when a patient leaves the ward with severe Parkinsonism, which can persist for several months. Under such circumstances, very few patients will be motivated to continue with long-acting medication, even if their psychosis has resolved.

Paliperidone and olanzapine in depot form are given in loading doses, resulting in a more rapid antipsychotic effect.

The older long-acting depot antipsychotics were introduced in an era before it was appreciated that there is a therapeutic window of dopamine D_2 receptor blockade [144]. As a result, the older depots (e.g. haloperidol, flupentixol) can be prescribed across a wide range of doses, despite the absence of any scientific rationale for very high doses. The newer long-acting depots (e.g. paliperidone, aripiprazole) are licenced within a narrower dose range. They also come with more rigid, one-size fits all instructions for initiation, which inevitably means that some patients develop Parkinsonism and akathisia.

Over-medication can cause Parkinsonism and akathisia. Careful dosing is needed when initiating a potent antipsychotic, such as haloperidol decanoate. It is important to keep in mind that these adverse effects also occur with newer depots. Thus,

CHAPTER 3

Table 3.8 Long-acting depot preparations.

Drug	Time to peak plasma concentration (d)	British National Formulary (BNF) Dose range (mg)	Time to steady state (wk)	Half-life (d)	Admin. interval
Aripiprazole (Abilify maintena)	5–7	200–400	12	30–46	Monthly

The tolerability of oral aripiprazole should be assessed before depot aripiprazole is initiated.
Oral aripiprazole supplementation is necessary for 14 days both sides of the first depot injection.
Aripiprazole depot can be administered into the deltoid muscle.
Concomitant inhibitors of CYP3A4 OR CYP2D6, reduce dose of aripiprazole depot.
Weight gain 0/+.
■ Dose-related akathisia.

Drug	Time to peak plasma concentration (d)	British National Formulary (BNF) Dose range (mg)	Time to steady state (wk)	Half-life (d)	Admin. interval
Aripiprazole Lauroxil (Aristada)	5–6	441 or 662	16	29–35	Monthly
		882			6-Weekly

The tolerability of oral aripiprazole should be assessed before Aristada is initiated.
Oral aripiprazole for 21 days in conjunction with first Aristada injection.
Only the smallest dose of Aristada can be administered into the deltoid muscle.
Concomitant inhibitors of CYP3A4 OR CYP2D6, reduce dose of Aristada.
Weight gain 0/+.
■ ! Dose-related akathisia.

Drug	Time to peak plasma concentration (d)	British National Formulary (BNF) Dose range (mg)	Time to steady state (wk)	Half-life (d)	Admin. interval
1-Monthly Paliperidone Palmitate PP-1M	13	25–150	—	25–49	Monthly

Immediate, continuous release.
No need for oral supplementation.
Initiation regime: 150 mg on day 1 and 100 mg on day 8, both administered into the deltoid muscle. Thereafter once monthly injections administered into either the deltoid or gluteal muscles.
Advantage of non-hepatic metabolism, but avoid in renal impairment (creatinine clearance <50 ml min⁻¹).
■ Dose-related motor side effects.

Drug	Time to peak plasma concentration (d)	British National Formulary (BNF) Dose range (mg)	Time to steady state (wk)	Half-life (d)	Admin. interval
3-Monthly Paliperidone Palmitate PP-3M	23–34	175 263 350 525	—	60–90	3-Monthly

Only recommended for patients treated with PP-1M for at least 4 months.
1st dose of PP-3M given at scheduled time of PP-1M (±1 week).
A dose of 3.5 × the last dose of PP-1M should be given.
Subsequent doses are given every 3 months (±2 weeks).
Avoid in renal impairment (creatinine clearance <50 ml min⁻¹).
Administered into either the deltoid or gluteal muscles.
■ Dose-related motor side effects.

Drug	Time to peak plasma concentration (d)	British National Formulary (BNF) Dose range (mg)	Time to steady state (wk)	Half-life (d)	Admin. interval
Flupentixol decanoate	7	Typical range 50 mg every 4 weeks to 300 mg every 2 weeks. (*Max 400 mg wk⁻¹*)	3–6	17	2–4 weeks

Table 3.8 (Continued)

Drug	Time to peak plasma concentration (d)	British National Formulary (BNF) Dose range (mg)	Time to steady state (wk)	Half-life (d)	Admin. interval
Test dose: 20 mg, then after at least 7 days: 20–40 mg at intervals of 2–4 weeks. Lower propensity for sedation. ■ Dose-related motor side effects.					
Zuclopenthixol decanoate	4–7	200–600 (*Max 600 mg wk⁻¹*)	8	7–19	1–4 weeks
Test dose: 100 mg, then after at least 7 days: 200–500 mg at intervals of 1–4 weeks. ■ Dose-related motor side effects.					
Fluphenazine decanoate	0.5–1	12.5–100	3	14	2–5 weeks
Test dose: 6.25–12.5 mg, then after 4–7 days: 12.5–100 mg repeated at intervals of 14–35 days. ■ Dose-related motor side effects.					
Risperidone Microspheres	28	25–50	8	4–6	2 weekly
After a single IM dose, the release of risperidone begins in week 3 and subsides by week 7. Oral risperidone supplementation is necessary for 3 weeks after the first depot injection. Risperidone depot can be administered into the deltoid muscle. ■ Dose-related motor side effects.					
Haloperidol decanoate	3–9	12.5–300	8–12	21	4 weekly
■ Dose-related motor side effects Initial dose typically 50 mg every 4 weeks. Max 300 mg every 4 weeks. Haloperidol depot can be administered into the deltoid muscle.					
Olanzapine Pamoate	2–4	150–300	8–12	14–30	2–4 weeks
Immediate, continuous release. No need for oral supplementation. ■ Post-injection syndrome (0.07% of injections). After each injection, patients should be observed for the symptoms and signs of olanzapine overdose in a healthcare facility by appropriately qualified personnel for at least three hours.					

Source: Data from electronic medicines compendium (EMC). www.medicines.org.uk/emc.

paliperidone can cause Parkinsonism, and depot aripiprazole is prone to inducing akathisia, a particularly unpleasant side effect [145, 146].

Selection of formulations and doses should occur in the context of a full history, with particular emphasis on previous response to antipsychotic treatment, previous dystonia, Parkinsonism or akathisia. The possibility of drug interactions should be assessed (Appendix 1). Starting doses of depot antipsychotic are lower in the elderly.

3.7.1 Clozapine

Clozapine is the treatment of choice for treatment-resistant schizophrenia. After six weeks of clozapine treatment about 30% of treatment-resistant patients will have

CHAPTER 3

improved. By six months of treatment between 60% and 70% of formerly treatment-resistant patients will have improved [147, 148].

It is prudent to distinguish between genuine treatment resistance and apparent treatment resistance arising from poor adherence to treatment. Approximately 40% of patients referred to the specialist clozapine clinic at the Maudsley as treatment resistant were in fact poorly adherent to antipsychotic medication as indicated by plasma drug monitoring [149].

Clozapine has a specific anti-suicidal effect. Approximately 5–10% of patients with schizophrenia will eventually complete suicide. Clozapine treatment markedly reduces the suicide rate in schizophrenia [150, 151].

Clozapine has a specific effect to reduce aggression and violence [148, 152].

Clozapine does not exhibit motor side effects. It can be used as a treatment for psychosis occurring in patients with Parkinson's disease [153]. Clozapine can be an effective treatment for tardive dyskinesia [154].

Providing a trial of clozapine for an individual patient can be challenging, but efforts to overcome the barriers and find solutions are worthwhile. Many patients who were severely disabled by chronic psychosis or negative syndrome schizophrenia have had their lives transformed by clozapine [155].

During the initiation phase, in which the dose of drug is gradually titrated, there is a need to monitor blood pressure, heart-rate and temperature for at least three hours following each dose, morning and evening. Ideally, monitoring should last 28 days.

The ideal care package is the initiation of clozapine as an in-patient or day-patient, but these resources are often unavailable for patients in modern psychiatric services.

The initiation of clozapine in the community is feasible but places significant time demands on staff managing a caseload of over 20 other patients [156]. If available, HTTs can be very helpful in sharing the monitoring requirements, particularly for the evening doses.

Some NHS trusts have set up a specialised central service to initiate community treatment. The goal is to reduce the average four-year delay before treatment-resistant patients access a trial of clozapine [157].

The most severely disabled schizophrenic patients can make a significant recovery with clozapine. However, such patients may be so disorganised, apathetic, impoverished, and isolated, that clozapine treatment is only feasible when provided alongside a package of rehabilitative support [158, 159]. It is important that this resource is not diverted away from the most disabled schizophrenic patients.

Patients can be reluctant to start clozapine because of the need for blood tests. However, it is worthwhile revisiting discussions. It might also be helpful for patients to meet others who have experienced the benefits of clozapine, following many years of suffering, disability and hitherto ineffective treatment.

3.7.2 Clozapine resistant psychosis

A proportion of patients fail to respond to a trial of clozapine (8–10 months) at adequate plasma concentrations (>0.35–$0.5\,\text{mg}\,\text{l}^{-1}$). There are various augmentation strategies, although it should be borne in mind that the evidence comes from relatively small trials, and case series, rather than from definitive phase III trials.

- Add in lamotrigine (aim for 200 mg d^{-1}). A meta-analysis of five randomised controlled trials (RCTs) of 10–24 weeks duration, involving a total of 161 patients showed that lamotrigine augmentation was beneficial for positive and negative symptoms [160].
- Add in topiramate. A recent meta-analysis of 16 RCTs involving 934 patients showed that adjunctive topiramate is effective for psychotic symptoms and weight reduction [161]. Side effects include attention/concentration difficulties, psychomotor slowing and paraesthesia.
- Add in 2nd antipsychotic: [162] This is a relatively common practice [163].
- *Clozapine + aripiprazole*
  In a recent meta-analysis (*n* = 347), the addition of aripiprazole (8–24 weeks) was beneficial for body weight and low-density lipoprotein (LDL) cholesterol, and there was a strong trend for improvement in psychotic symptoms, with the downside of increased rates of agitation/akathisia [164].
- *Clozapine + sulpiride*
  A meta-analysis of three RCTs suggested that the addition of sulpiride improved hypersalivation and body weight, with the downside of more movement disorder and hyperprolactinemia. The addition of sulpiride had no effect on global state or relapse rates [165].
- Add in memantine (20 mg d^{-1}). Two small RCTs provide support for this approach, although there are inconsistencies. The more recent trial (*n* = 52, 12 weeks) found small-moderate benefits for negative symptoms but not positive symptoms [166]. An earlier trial (*n* = 21, 12 weeks) reported benefits for positive and negative symptoms [167].
- Add in omega-3 fatty acids. A small-scale study (*n* = 31) reported benefits for the addition of ethyl-eicosapentaenoate 2 g d^{-1} on triglyceride levels and psychotic symptoms [168].
- Electroconvulsive therapy (ECT). A number of small-scale studies have suggested that ECT may be an efficacious and safe treatment for clozapine resistant psychosis [169]. For example, in an eight-week trial (*n* = 39) the addition of ECT led to clinical improvement in 50% of previously clozapine-resistant patients [170].

If there are mood symptoms as part of the overall clinical picture, consider antidepressants or mood stabilisers [104].

3.7.3   Side effects of clozapine

Side effects can be recorded systematically with the Glasgow Antipsychotic side-effects scale for clozapine [171]. Side effects account for the majority clozapine discontinuations, particularly in the first few months of treatment. Clinicians should be alert to the management of side effects to minimise potentially avoidable discontinuations [172].

Clozapine is associated with adverse metabolic effects that sometimes deter clinicians from prescribing it. However, on average, patients with schizophrenia who are treated with clozapine actually have a greater life expectancy than those treated with other antipsychotic medications or those who are untreated [173].

3.7.3.1 Sedation

Clozapine has sedative properties because of its high affinity for the histamine H_1 receptor. Sedation is the most common reason for discontinuation of clozapine [172].

3.7.3.2 Pyrexia

The initiation of clozapine is associated with a benign, transient pyrexia in about 10–50% of patients [174]. However, pyrexia in patients taking clozapine should always be investigated as it can be associated with neutropenia/agranulocytosis, myocarditis and neuroleptic malignant syndrome (NMS).

If temp >38 °C: Examine for infection, check full blood count (FBC), C-reactive protein (CRP), troponin, creatine kinase (CK). Exclude neutropenia/agranulocytosis, myocarditis and NMS. Paracetamol, slow titration or temporary discontinuation/re-challenge [175, 104].

3.7.3.3 Postural hypotension

Clozapine can cause orthostatic hypotension, which manifests as dizziness upon standing. The cause is reduced vascular tone stemming from blockade of α_1-adrenoceptors on blood vessels [176]. Clozapine has markedly higher affinity for the α_1-adrenoceptor than the dopamine D_2 receptor. Postural hypotension is a feature of the early stages of treatment and usually shows tolerance over several weeks. In young patients, with careful dose titration, it is rarely an issue.

3.7.3.4 Tachycardia

Clozapine can increase the heart rate (tachycardia). In normal physiology, the heart pacemaker is tonically inhibited by the vagus nerve and accelerated by sympathetic nerve activity. Clozapine causes tachycardia by blocking the vagal 'brake' (M_2-muscarinic effect) while boosting the sympathetic 'accelerator' (α_2-adrenoceptor effect) [176].

Clozapine-elicited tachycardia occurs in about 25% of patients during dose titration [177]. Tachycardia is related to the speed of titration [178]. In most patients, tachycardia shows tolerance over a period of weeks but may persist in some.

Treatment with a cardio-selective β-blocker such as bisoprolol is usually very effective against tachycardia, although an eye has to be kept out for hypotension [179]. Ivabradine is an alternative [180].

- Tachycardia can also be a symptom of myocarditis.

3.7.4 Myocarditis: inflammation of heart muscle

Estimates of the risk of myocarditis from clozapine treatment vary widely, ranging from 1 in 1 000 to as high as 1 in 30 [181]. The majority of cases (80%) emerge in the first month of starting clozapine. The risk of myocarditis is not dose related. Guidelines are as follows [182].

The clinical picture includes, fever, tachycardia, chest pain, ↑ respiratory rate (>20 min^{-1}), ↓ systolic BP (<100 mmHg), ↑ CRP >100 mg l^{-1}, ↑ troponin >2 × upper normal limit, and eosinophilia.

CRP and troponin should be assessed at baseline, alongside an ECG. (*Baseline echocardiography has also been suggested* [182] *although there is doubt that any benefit outweighs the considerable cost of screening* [183].

CRP and troponin should be assessed weekly for 28 days.

If symptoms of infectious illness OR tachycardia >120 bpm or rise >30 bpm OR CRP 50–100 mg l^{-1} OR troponin elevated to <2 × upper normal limit:

Continue clozapine with daily troponin and CRP until abnormality resolves.

- If troponin elevated to >2 × upper normal limit OR CRP >100 mg l^{-1}:

Cease clozapine.
Consult cardiologist.
Echocardiogram +/– cardiac MRI.

3.7.5 Cardiomyopathy: impaired function of heart muscle

Cardiomyopathy is less common than myocarditis, and its onset is slower, typically emerging many months after initiating clozapine. The symptoms are those of heart failure: dyspnoea and palpitations [184]. Clozapine cessation and referral to a cardiologist is required.

3.7.6 The effects of clozapine at muscarinic M_1–M_4 acetylcholine receptors

Clozapine has a unique pharmacology at muscarinic acetylcholine receptors. There is persuasive evidence that agonism at M_4 receptors is associated with an antipsychotic effect [185].

In isolated cells, clozapine is a partial agonist at M_1, M_2, M_3, and M_4 receptors [186, 187], but body organs are far more complex, dynamic systems. The general rule is that if a cholinergic nerve such as the vagus is actively communicating with tissue, clozapine behaves as an antagonist but in the absence of signalling from the nerve, clozapine exerts a prolonged low-level stimulation of the tissue.

3.7.6.1 *Hyper-Salivation*

Secretion from salivary glands is driven, in part, by cholinergic nerves which act on M_3, M_4, and M_1 receptors [188]. Clozapine can stimulate the salivary glands (M_3/M_4/M_1) causing bothersome drooling at night in at least one-third of patients [189].

Anticholinergics are the usual treatment: hyoscine tablets sucked 0.3 mg up to tds or hyoscine patch 1.5 mg in 72 hours; pirenzepine 25–100 mg d^{-1}; glycopyrrolate 1 mg bd. Glycopyrrolate is non-CNS penetrant [104].

In a recent trial, metoclopramide (10–30 mg d^{-1}) was shown to be effective in two-thirds of patients and was well tolerated [190].

3.7.6.2   *Nocturnal enuresis*

Muscle contraction in the bladder is driven by cholinergic nerves acting at M_3 and M_2 receptors, whereas tone in the urethral sphincter is maintained by adrenergic nerves at acting at α_1-receptors [188]. Clozapine can stimulate bladder contraction (M_3/M_2) and relax the urethral sphincter (α_1). As a consequence, about one in five patients on clozapine experience night time bed-wetting. In the majority of cases, enuresis shows tolerance but is clearly a source of distress [191].

Exclude diabetes mellitus, diabetes insipidus, and nocturnal seizures.
Small-case series support the use of anticholinergics: e.g. oxybutynin 5 mg; and desmo-
pressin but watch for hyponatremia [191].

3.7.6.3   *Reduced gastrointestinal motility*

Cholinergic nerves stimulate gastrointestinal motility via M_3 and M_2 receptors [188]. In the gut clozapine behaves as an antagonist, inhibiting gut motility.

Clozapine can inhibit gastromotility at all levels of the gastrointestinal tract, constituting a risk for gastroparesis, choking, aspiration pneumonia, constipation, and ileus [192].

Clozapine causes constipation in about one-third of patients, but may go unrecognised [193].

- Examine for as well as ask about constipation (Patient reports on their own may be unreliable). Treatment: Stimulant laxatives (Bisacodyl, senna, picolax, glycerol suppositories, docusate sodium) and osmotic laxatives (Movicol, laxido, lactulose) [193]. Docusate sodium is also a stool softener.
    Avoid bulk forming laxatives
- Severe constipation can be life-threatening through bowel obstruction, perforation and sepsis [193].

3.7.7   Weight-gain and type II diabetes

See Sections 6.1 and 6.2.

3.7.8   Neutropenia and agranulocytosis

Neutropenia is defined as a circulating neutrophil count of $<1.5 \times 10^9$ l^{-1}. Neutropenia occurs in 2.9% of clozapine treated patients [194].

Agranulocytosis is defined as a circulating neutrophil count of $<0.5 \times 10^9$ l^{-1}. Agranulocytosis occurs in 0.8% of clozapine treated patients. Eighty per cent of cases emerge in the first 18 weeks [194].

Blood monitoring of white cell and neutrophil counts is mandatory. This should be done weekly for 18 weeks, then fortnightly for 1 year, then monthly thereafter.

Blood thresholds differ between the USA and the UK. In the USA, patients are required to have a minimum neutrophil count of 1.5×10^9 l^{-1} to initiate clozapine. In the UK, white cell and neutrophil counts are categorised as green, amber, and red as shown in Table 3.9.

Table 3.9 Clozapine and neutrophil counts in the UK.

	Green	Amber	Red
White Cell count ($\times 10^9$ l^{-1})	≥3.5	<3.5	<3.0
Neutrophils count ($\times 10^9$ l^{-1})	≥2.0	<2.0	<1.5
	Continue clozapine	Twice weekly blood monitoring until a green result is obtained	Stop clozapine Daily blood monitoring Monitor for infection - Hospital admission

3.7.8.1   Benign ethnic neutropenia

Many people of African descent and some groups from the middle east have naturally occurring low neutrophil counts without any consequences for infection. This is known as benign ethnic neutropenia (BEN) [195]. Before commencement of clozapine, BEN patients have neutrophil counts around the risk threshold and this is persistent [196].

In BEN patients, the amber and red thresholds are reduced by 0.5. This can allow BEN patients to access clozapine treatment, and reduce unnecessary blood tests [197]. Some patients with BEN have been able to access clozapine by having their white cell and neutrophils counts increased by lithium treatment (Li$^+$ levels >0.4 mmol l^{-1}). The mechanism underlying this effect of lithium is unknown, but note that lithium has no protective effect on true clozapine-induced neutropenia or agranulocytosis [196].

3.7.8.2   Clozapine re-challenge

It is possible to re-challenge patients with clozapine after an episode of neutropenia. However, specialist psychiatric and haematological advice should be sought from the outset. Granulocyte-colony stimulating factor (GCS-F) can be used to stimulate the bone marrow although it probably does not protect against agranulocytosis. Clozapine-associated neutropenia can emerge more quickly and be more severe second time around [196].

Re-challenge should not be attempted after an episode of clozapine-induced agranulocytosis.

3.7.9   Lowered seizure threshold

Clozapine is associated with an increased risk of seizures [198]. A common practice is to begin prophylactic anticonvulsant at doses above 600 mg d^{-1}, but the rationale for this has been debated [199]. The risk of seizures increases linearly over the dose range. There is no threshold dose or plasma level, however, plasma levels of clozapine ≥1.3 mg/L are associated with a very substantial risk of seizures. Close clinical monitoring, measurement of plasma levels, alertness to drug interactions and dose adjustment is recommended [199]. Where anticonvulsants are deemed necessary for secondary prevention, valproate and lamotrigine can be used, although valproate increases the risk of weight gain and is contraindicated in women of child-bearing age [199]. Carbamazepine should be avoided because of the risk of bone marrow suppression.

Chapter 4

Bipolar disorder

4.1 Diagnosis of bipolar

There can be a delay of around 5–10 years and much suffering before bipolar patients receive the correct diagnosis [200].

Periods of hypomania ('mini-mania') may be missed in a history dominated by recurrent depression, leading to an incorrect diagnosis of unipolar depression and frustrated responses to antidepressants and talking therapy. The correct diagnosis (bipolar II), finally permits appropriate pharmacological treatment [201].

A recent trend in UK early-intervention services is the tendency to categorise a manic episode within the *catch-all* term unspecified psychosis (ICD10 F29). The utility of unspecified psychosis is that it provides a holding category until a more complete clinical picture manifests, but the risk is that the correct diagnosis (bipolar I) is missed, leading to errors in treatment planning.

Bipolar disorders are usually lifelong [33] The one-size fits all category of ICD10 F29 unspecified psychosis often comes with advice about stopping medication after 12–18 months, but in the natural history of bipolar, 12–18 months is a very short timeframe [202]. Such pharmacological advice usually turns out to be unhelpful for bipolar patients, even although their initial recovery can be impressive.

Drug and alcohol misuse is common in people with bipolar disorder (lifetime risk of 44% and 48% respectively) and can cloud the clinical picture [203, 204]. Comorbid addiction worsens the clinical course and increases the risk of suicide [205, 206]. Cocaine, amphetamines, mephedrone, high-potency cannabis and synthetic cannabinoids can elicit acute hypomania and mania. In the opposite direction of causality, hypomania and mania can drive pleasure-seeking, risk-taking and problematic drug use. Cause and effect relationships can only be established on an individual basis, paying close attention to the clinical picture over time [207].

The bipolar spectrum shares instability of mood with borderline personality disorder, as a common feature. Discriminating features are that borderline tends to have no

Advanced Prescribing in Psychosis, First Edition. Paul Morrison, David M. Taylor and Phillip McGuire.
© 2020 John Wiley & Sons Ltd. Published 2020 by John Wiley & Sons Ltd.

clear-cut onset, that impulsivity is chronic rather than episodic, that mood shifts are more frequent (and dysphoric/angry rather than depressed/elated) and that suicidal gestures and deliberate self-harm are much more common. Borderline patients have specific difficulties in cooperation. Both conditions are heritable, although bipolar genetics receive much more attention. Illness severity is also associated with early abuse and neglect, but this receives particular emphasis in borderline cases [208, 209].

4.2   Treatment of mania

Prescribing decisions should be made in relation to individual patient factors. Consideration is given to possible organic causation, drugs/alcohol, physical health, and pregnancy [210]. If mania occurs within bipolar disorder then it is essential to review the pattern over time, adherence and response to treatment, and any recent change to treatment.

Note:
Antidepressants can trigger mania [211].
In mania, antidepressants should be tapered and stopped [212].
Abrupt lithium discontinuation can trigger an acute mania [213].

In the era before pharmacotherapy, mania could persist for months. Sedative hypnotics could provide brief respite, but the mania would resume on wakening. Talking therapies are unfeasible. Lithium was the first anti-manic agent, and has an effect within approximately four days.

Mania responds to lithium, valproate, carbamazepine, and dopamine D_2 antipsychotics [212] (Table 4.1). The antipsychotics have a relatively quick onset of action [214].

Currently, atypical antipsychotics are regarded as first-line treatments for mania [214].

The addition of a benzodiazepine can be helpful for over-activity, agitation, insomnia, and excitement [212].

A proportion of manic patients may not respond to treatment with a single drug. Combinations have additional efficacy over and above monotherapy [212].

Antipsychotic + valproate OR lithium [215, 216].
Antipsychotic + valproate + lithium [217].

When lithium or valproate are used, plasma drug monitoring is required.

Lithium can be increased to maximum plasma levels of up to 1.0 mmol l-1 [212].
Valproate can be increased to maximum plasma levels of up to 125 mg l-1 [104].

For treatment resistant mania, clozapine is effective [218–220].
Electroconvulsive therapy (ECT) is effective for treatment-resistant mania [221].

4.3   Treatment of bipolar depression

The appropriate way to treat the depressive phase of bipolar disorder is controversial [33]. It is often considered difficult to treat with antidepressants (i.e. drugs developed and tested in unipolar depression) [211]. Monotherapy is not recommended in bipolar

Table 4.1 Drug treatment of bipolar disorder.

Drug	Mechanism	Upside	Downside
'Mood stabiliser' class			
Lithium carbonate Starting dose: 400mg nocte. (200mg in elderly) See Appendix 4 for plasma level monitoring.	↑ Neurotrophic signals: AKT stimulation GSK3β inhibition Inositol depletion Na⁺ channel blocker	Effective in acute mania. Especially effective in reducing relapse to the manic pole. Reduces the suicide rate by >80% Reduces relapse to the depressive pole.	Narrow therapeutic index. Blood testing needed. Weight-gain. Polyuria. Tremor Thyroid and parathyroid dysfunction. Rebound mania on abrupt discontinuation. Less effective in rapid cycling.

Plasma levels of 0.6–0.8 mmol l⁻¹ are usually needed for effective prophylaxis.
In mania plasma levels can be increased up to 1.0 mmol l⁻¹.
- Toxicity: Plasma levels of 1.5 mmol l⁻¹.
- Nonsteroidal non-inflammatory drugs (NSAIDs), angiotensin-converting enzyme (ACE) inhibitors, diuretics, steroids, tetracyclines can ↑ Li⁺ plasma levels.
- Avoid dehydration.
Lithium and renal failure? Population rate, 1 in 500: On lithium 1 in 200.
No risk of lithium for renal malignancy.
– Lithium and fetal heart valve abnormalities? Population rate 1 in 20 000; On lithium in pregnancy 1 in 1000–2000.

Drug	Mechanism	Upside	Downside
Valproate Starting dose: 500 mg d⁻¹ Typical dose: 1000–2000 mg d⁻¹ See Appendix 1 for interactions and kinetics. See Appendix 4 for plasma level monitoring.	↑ DNA transcription: HDAC inhibition. ↑ Neurotrophic signals: GSK3β inhibition prolongs Na + channel inactivation ? ↑ GABA signalling	Effective in acute mania. Probably reduces relapse to the manic pole. Probably reduces relapse to the depressive pole. Anti-convulsant	Less effective than lithium in the maintenance phase. Weight-gain. Tremor. Nausea. Teratogenicity.

- Contraindicated in females of childbearing age, unless the conditions of Prevent – the valproate pregnancy prevention programme are fulfilled https://assets. publishing.service.gov.uk/government/uploads/system/uploads/attachment_data/file/708850/123683_Valproate_HCP_Booklet_DR15.pdf
- Contraindicated in pregnancy in bipolar.
Folic acid supplements do not guarantee protection against neural tube defects.

Drug	Mechanism	Upside	Downside
Lamotrigine Starting dose: 25 mg d⁻¹ for two weeks. Typical dose: 200 mg d⁻¹ See Appendix 1 for interactions and kinetics. See Appendix 4 for plasma level monitoring.	Na⁺ channel blocker Ca²⁺channel blocker ? ↓ glutamate signalling	Reduces relapse to the depressive pole. Bipolar depression. Weight neutral. Well tolerated. Anti-convulsant.	Six-week titration of dose. Ineffective in acute mania. Ineffective for preventing relapse to mania.

(Continued)

Table 4.1 (Continued)

Drug	Mechanism	Upside	Downside
Skin rash. Serious skin rashes including Stevens-Johnson approx. 1 in 1 000. Pregnancy. No significant increased rates of major congenital malformation above background rate. Risk of cleft palate? Population rate 1 in 700. On lamotrigine in pregnancy 1 in 550.			
Carbamazepine Oral 400–1200 mg d^{-1} See Appendix 1 for interactions and kinetics. See Appendix 4 for plasma level monitoring.	prolongs Na+channel inactivation ? ↑ GABA signalling	Effective in acute mania (but not used 1st line)	Less effective than lithium in the maintenance phase (3rd line use). Dose-related central nervous system (CNS) side-effects, ataxia, diplopia. Nausea. Allergic skin reactions. Leucopenia. Multiple drug interactions (Appendix 1: Pharmacokinetics of selected psychotropics) Teratogenicity.

- AVOID carbamazepine in pregnancy. High risk of neural tube defects.
- Not recommended in females of childbearing age.
- Folic acid supplements do not guarantee protection against neural tube defects.
- Carbamazepine can result in the failure of oral contraceptives containing oestrogen and/or progesterone.

Antipsychotic class

Drug	Mechanism	Upside	Downside
Aripiprazole oral 5–30 mg d^{-1}	D$_2$ partial agonist 5HT$_{2A}$ antagonist 5HT$_{1A}$ partial agonist 5HT$_7$ antagonist 5HT$_{2C}$ partial agonist α$_2$ antagonist	Effective in acute mania. Reduces relapse to the manic pole. Weight gain 0/+. Available as a depot.	Akathisia. Nausea. Insomnia.
Quetiapine Starting dose: 100mg. oral 150–750 mg d^{-1} (in mania max. is 800 mg d^{-1})	H$_1$ antagonist α$_1$ antagonist D$_2$ antagonist *at higher doses*	Effective in bipolar depression. Effective in acute mania. Reduces relapse to the manic pole. Reduces relapse to the depressive pole.	Sedation. Weight gain++ Dyslipidemia. Hyperglycemia. Postural hypotension.
Norquetiapine	*5HT$_{2C}$ antagonist* *NET inhibitor* *M$_1$ antagonist*		

Drug	Mechanism	Upside	Downside
Olanzapine oral 5–20 mg d^{-1}	H_1 antagonist $5HT_{2A}$ antagonist $5HT_{2C}$ inverse agonist D_2 antagonist M_1-M_5 antagonist	Effective in acute mania. Olanzapine+fluoxetine in combination effective in acute depression. Reduces relapse to the manic pole.	Sedation. Weight gain+++ Dyslipidemia. Hyperglycemia. Risk of type II diabetes. (Depot preparation available, but problematic to use in routine practice).
Risperidone Starting dose: 2 mg oral 2–16 mg d^{-1}	$5HT_2$ inverse agonist D_2 antagonist $5HT_7$ antagonist α_1 antagonist $5HT_{2C}$ inverse agonist H_1 antagonist α_2 antagonist	Effective in acute mania. Reduces relapse to the manic pole. Available as a depot.	EPSEs Risk of tardive dyskinesia. High prolactin. Weight gain+ Erectile dysfunction. Postural hypotension.
Lurasidone oral 18.5–148 mg d^{-1}	$5HT_7$ antagonist D_2 antagonist $5HT_{2A}$ antagonist α_2 antagonist $5HT_{1A}$ partial agonist	Effective in bipolar depression. Probably effective in acute mania. Probably reduces relapse to the manic pole. Probably reduces relapse to the depressive pole. Weight gain 0/+.	Akathisia. Sedation.
Clozapine starting dose: 12.5 mg usual maintenance: 200–450 mg d^{-1} max: 900 mg d^{-1} guided by plasma levels. Target >0.35–0.5 mgl^{-1} (Trough).	H1 antagonist α_1 antagonist $5HT_{2A}$ antagonist $5HT_{2C}$ inverse agonist M_1-M_5 partial agonist $5HT_7$ antagonist D_2 antagonist *at higher doses*	Efficacy in treatment-resistant mania.	Sedation. Weight gain+++ Dyslipidemia. Hyperglycemia. Risk of type II diabetes. Tachycardia. Hyper-salivation. Need for blood tests. Rebound psychosis. Myocarditis. Constipation.

(Continued)

Table 4.1 (Continued)

Drug	Mechanism	Upside	Downside
Cariprazine Starting dose: 1.5 mg d^{-1} target dose: 3–6 mg d^{-1}	D$_2$ partial agonist 5HT$_{1A}$ partial agonist 5HT$_{2A}$ antagonist H$_1$ antagonist 5HT$_{2C}$ inverse agonist at higher doses	Effective in acute mania. Probably reduces relapse to the manic pole. Maintained efficacy with missed doses because of very long half-life of cariprazine and its active metabolite. Weight gain 0/+.	Akathisia EPSEs Insomnia
Asenapine Sub-lingual 5 mg b.d. – 10 mg b.d	5HT$_{2C}$ antagonist 5HT$_{2A}$ antagonist 5HT$_7$ antagonist H$_1$ antagonist H$_2$ antagonist α_1 antagonist α_2 antagonist D$_2$ antagonist 5HT$_{1A}$ partial agonist	Effective in acute mania. Probably reduces relapse to the manic pole.	Sedation EPSEs Weight gain+ Oral hypoesthesia Postural hypotension.
Ziprasidone 20–80 mg b.d.	5HT$_{2A}$ antagonist 5HT$_{2C}$ partial agonist D$_2$ antagonist 5HT$_{1A}$ partial agonist 5HT$_7$ antagonist α_1 antagonist H$_1$ antagonist	Effective in acute mania. Probably reduces relapse to the manic pole. Weight gain 0/+	↑ QTc by >20 msec Insomnia EPSEs Risk of tardive dyskinesia

Key:

D$_2$ antagonist – antipsychotic, high prolactin, motor side effects

α_1 antagonist – postural hypotension, efficacy against nightmares in post-traumatic stress disorder (PTSD).

α_2 antagonist – antidepressant

NET inhibitor (*noradrenaline re-uptake inhibition*) – antidepressant.

H$_1$ antagonist – sedation, weight gain.

5HT$_{1A}$ partial agonist – anxiolytic.

5HT$_{2A}$ antagonist – antipsychotic activity?? inhibits Parkinsonism? pro-cognitive??

5HT$_{2C}$ inverse agonist/antagonist – weight gain.

5HT$_{2C}$ antagonist – antidepressant?

5HT$_7$ antagonist – antidepressant?

M$_1$–M$_5$ partial agonist/antagonist – inhibits Parkinsonism, constipation, urinary retention/incontinence, blurred vision, dry mouth (antagonist)/hyper-salivation (partial agonist), tachycardia.

Source: Data from: Psychoactive Drug Screening Program (PDSP) database (University of North Carolina, USA).Electronic medicines compendium (EMC). www.medicines.org.uk/emc.

I patients because it can trigger a switch to mania in ~10–25% of patients [33]. The risk of switching is highest for dual serotonin/noradrenaline re-uptake inhibitors (venlafaxine, duloxetine, tricyclics). Concomitant mood stabilisers or antipsychotics reduce the risk of switching [211].

Although they are mentioned in the UK NICE guidelines, there is little evidence to support the use of talking therapies for the treatment of bipolar depression [222].

Effective pharmacotherapies for bipolar depression have emerged (Table 4.1). Recent trials have demonstrated that the following pharmacological treatments are effective with an effect size in the moderate range:

Quetiapine [223]
Lurasidone [224]
Olanzapine + fluoxetine combination [225].

Lamotrigine is effective when added to quetiapine for acute bipolar depression [226]. Monotherapy trials of lamotrigine in bipolar depression were poorly conducted, and misleadingly suggest a small effect size. Lamotrigine is particularly useful in the maintenance phase because of a low side effect burden. Lamotrigine reduces the chances of a relapse and re-admission for depression. It may be particularly useful as monotherapy in bipolar II disorder where switch to hypomania is relatively low risk. Lamotrigine is currently under-used compared with antidepressants in the UK [227].

Quetiapine is regarded as a first-line treatment for bipolar depression. Lurasidone has similar efficacy and the advantage of being less sedative and relatively weight neutral, but it is currently more expensive and less clinical experience has accrued.

ECT is effective for bipolar depression. In treatment-resistant bipolar depression, where there is a high suicide risk or pregnancy, ECT should be considered [228].

4.4   The maintenance phase of bipolar: relapse prevention

Following the index episode, an individual has a 10% chance of avoiding a relapse over their lifetime [229, 230]. At one and three years, the chances of avoiding a relapse are, approximately, less than 50% and 30% respectively [231]. Relapse can be either manic, depressive or mixed, with depression being most common [231].

Many patients suffer from multiple relapses [232]. Successive episodes last longer, become more resistant to treatment, cognitive impairment can emerge and the suicide rate increases.

The risk of completed suicide in bipolar is between 20–30 × higher than in the general population. Lithium has been shown to markedly reduce the suicide rate in bipolar patients [233, 234].

The British association of psychopharmacology (BAP) guidelines recommend lithium as a first-line treatment for maintenance therapy in bipolar I, with the caveat that patients need to show a willingness to adhere, as swift discontinuation can trigger a manic relapse [212] (Table 4.1).

Maintenance pharmacotherapy significantly reduces a patient's chances of relapse [235].

CHAPTER 4

Large clinical trials have shown that antipsychotics and mood stabilisers clearly reduce relapse rates. In the SPaRCLE trial [236], 1 200 patients were followed up over two years. Of those who were randomly allocated to placebo, less than 20% avoided a relapse. In contrast, those who were allocated to either the lithium group or the quetiapine group had a 60% chance of avoiding a relapse over the two years.

A Finnish study collected follow-up data on over 18 000 patients who had been hospitalised because of bipolar disorder. Over a period of seven years, patients treated with lithium or antipsychotics had lower rates of re-hospitalisation. Long-acting depot antipsychotics out-performed equivalent oral formulations in terms of re-hospitalisation [237].

Combination treatments outperform monotherapy in avoiding relapse [238]. Some patients may prefer this option as the consequences of another episode can be very severe.

A large trial followed 600 bipolar patients over two years. Patients treated with monotherapy (lithium or valproate) were compared with those treated with a combination (quetiapine + lithium or valproate). Those who were randomly allocated to monotherapy had a 60% chance of avoiding a manic or depressive episode. In contrast, those who were allocated to combination therapy had a 90% chance of avoiding mania, and an 80% chance of avoiding an episode of depression over the two years [239].

Residual mood symptoms at recovery predict relapse [231]. In modern psychiatric services bipolar patients are often discharged from hospital while still experiencing residual symptoms. There can then be a swift re-admission as things break down again. It is vital that patients are reviewed frequently by their community psychiatrist or by the home treatment team in the weeks following discharge. An episode of mania can take over 12 weeks to fully resolve.

When stability has returned, a package of psycho-education is vital. Ideally, over time, patients can develop expertise in managing their own condition [240].

As a general rule, bipolar patients recover insight upon recovery from a manic episode [241]. As health recovers bipolar patients recognise that they were mentally unwell in a prior depressive or manic episode. Even so, many patients find it difficult to accept the diagnosis of bipolar, especially in the early years. Understandably, there can be a reluctance to rely on managing one's mood with medication. It can take several episodes and much disruption before a patient makes the decision to take maintenance treatment.

Patients need to hear accurate information about relapse rates in bipolar, on and off medication, to be able to make an informed decision about their treatment.

A retrospective mood chart can identify patterns that predict relapse.

There are now a range of apps which can track energy levels, sleep, mood, and other indices of mental health over time [242], although it is recommended that patients and clinicians should exercise caution in selecting which app to use [243].

Insomnia and an increased pace of thinking are common relapse indicators, but quite often mania can emerge so quickly as to overwhelm insight. Some patients benefit from the security of having a small supply of a sedative at home. A z-drug or sedative antihistamine is ideal for this purpose [244].

4.5 Bipolar in females of childbearing age

Relapse rates in bipolar are high in the perinatal period, particularly in the first few months post-partum [245, 246]. For women with bipolar I, maintenance pharmaco-therapy during pregnancy increases the chance of staying well in the post-partum from 34% *off-medication* to 77% *on-medication* [247].

Forward planning is desirable, although approximately one-half of pregnancies are unplanned [33]. Ideally, a treatment plan should be discussed and chosen ahead of a future pregnancy. The risks of treatment versus non-treatment can be discussed, and the profile of individual drugs can be compared. The discussion should also encompass alcohol, tobacco, other substances, and folate [245].

Many patients with bipolar I discontinue their medication abruptly on finding out that they are pregnant. However, discontinuation of medication is associated with very high rates of recurrence during pregnancy. Those who stop treatment abruptly have only a 15% chance of remaining well versus a 63% chance for those who remain on treatment [248].

Prescribing decisions should be based on an individualised risk-benefit analysis rather than a one size fits all approach [245]. Factors are diagnosis, illness severity, the pattern of acute episodes and response to medication [245].

For women whose history of major mental illness is *exclusively limited* to the post-partum period, a suggested approach is to begin prophylactic treatment immediately after delivery [249].

4.5.1 Valproate and carbamazepine in females of childbearing age

Valproate is now contraindicated in females of childbearing age, unless the conditions of Prevent – the valproate pregnancy prevention programme are fulfilled. https://assets.publishing.service.gov.uk/government/uploads/system/uploads/attachment_data/file/708850/123683_Valproate_HCP_Booklet_DR15.pdf.

Valproate is contraindicated in pregnancy in bipolar.

AVOID carbamazepine. There is a high risk of neural tube defects and low IQ [33].

Carbamazepine can result in the failure of oral contraceptives containing oestrogen and/or progesterone.

4.5.2 Lithium in females of childbearing age

Current expert opinion is that the benefits of lithium in pregnancy outweigh the risks to the developing fetus. Indeed, specific risks to the fetus are not definitively established despite early case reports that continue to be misleadingly cited [250, 33]. The risk of the Ebstein heart valve abnormality in the population is 1 in 20 000. Exposure to lithium during pregnancy increases the risk to 1 in 1000–2000 [251].

The greater risk is relapse after childbirth. This may be manic or depressive and, when psychotic, may be associated tragically with infanticide [252]. Where lithium is clearly effective against a pattern of repeated manic episodes, it will also provide

CHAPTER 4

protection against post-partum illness. However, close monitoring of the mental state is always mandatory.

Closer plasma monitoring of lithium levels during pregnancy is advised. NICE recommends that lithium levels are checked every four weeks in pregnancy and weekly after week 36 weeks. (www.nice.org.uk/guidance/cg192)

Breast-feeding should be avoided in women taking lithium because of the risk of toxicity in the newborn.

4.5.3   Lamotrigine in females of childbearing age

Current expert opinion is that lamotrigine carries no significant risk for teratogenesis above the baseline population rate [253]. However, one paper reported an increased risk of cleft palate. Later studies did not replicate this finding. The most recent and largest study gives the following estimate of cleft palate: Population rate 1 in 700. On lamotrigine in pregnancy 1 in 550 (*note: between group differences did not reach statistical significance*) [254].

4.5.4   Antipsychotics in females of childbearing age

Available data suggests that the antipsychotic class is safe in pregnancy, carrying no significant risk for teratogenesis above the baseline population rate [255].

NICE cautions on the use of those antipsychotics which are associated with extreme weight-gain and which carry a risk for diabetes. Monitoring for gestational diabetes and an oral glucose tolerance test is recommended (www.nice.org.uk/guidance/cg192).

Compared to antipsychotic discontinuation, olanzapine, and quetiapine increase the risk of gestational diabetes by 1.6 × and 1.3 × respectively [256].

In the post-partum period women taking sedative antipsychotics should be warned of the risk of falling asleep in bed beside their babies.

Breast-feeding should be avoided in women taking clozapine.

The role of talking therapies in the treatment of psychosis

5.1 Psychoanalytical insights

Classic psychoanalytical theory dominated American psychiatry until the 1970s. With the success of psychopharmacology beginning in the 1950s, a paradigm shift was inevitable [257, 258].

Over time, psychoanalytical theory recognised that mental illness was shaped by actual interpersonal experiences in early life and not just by unconscious forces, a view that resonates with the modern idea of modifiable neural networks [259]. Epidemiological studies have subsequently confirmed that bio-psychosocial adversity during development predisposes to a range of psychiatric disorders, including psychotic illness [260, 261].

Psychoanalytical awareness is very important for teams caring for patients with psychotic illnesses. Analytical space can help avoid common errors, such as the tendency to collude with some patients in 'normalising' a previous psychotic breakdown as an 'understandable reaction to stress' [262].

5.2 Psychological treatments

Modern psychological treatments such as cognitive behavioural therapy (CBT) focus on surface mental content with no recourse to the unconscious. CBT is an effective treatment for moderate unipolar depression and for anxiety syndromes [263].

Initial work suggested that CBT benefitted the symptoms of the at-risk mental state but a recent meta-analysis was negative [264, 265]. Moreover, CBT does not decrease the transition to psychotic illness [266].
There was hope that CBT would also be effective for the core symptoms of schizophrenia. However, any added benefit of CBT on psychotic symptoms over and above that

Advanced Prescribing in Psychosis, First Edition. Paul Morrison, David M. Taylor and Phillip McGuire.
© 2020 John Wiley & Sons Ltd. Published 2020 by John Wiley & Sons Ltd.

from a supportive therapeutic relationship appears to be small, to the point of being undetectable in better designed trials [267–270].

For example, in a recent trial involving 220 patients, there was no advantage of CBT over treatment as usual on the positive or negative symptoms of schizophrenia [271].

A recent Cochrane review found that there were no advantages of CBT for schizophrenia over other '*less sophisticated*' psychological therapies in terms of positive and negative psychotic symptoms, relapse rates, re-hospitalisation or social functioning [267].

Compared to treatment as usual, CBT does not offer protection against relapse in schizophrenia or bipolar disorder [268, 273–275]. CBT is also ineffective for clozapine resistant schizophrenia [276].

Despite the disappointing results, NICE have set the following targets for community teams looking after patients with a first episode psychosis: CBT should be offered to all patients with first-episode psychosis. CBT should be delivered over at least 16 sessions.(www.nice.org.uk/guidance/qs80/resources/psychosis-and-schizophrenia-in-adults-pdf-2098901855941).

Psycho-education appears to have a beneficial effect in reducing the chances of relapse in bipolar disorder [277].

Family intervention (FI) is effective in reducing the chances of relapse in schizophrenia [272, 278].

Cognitive remediation therapy (CRT) appears to be effective for improving the cognitive symptoms of schizophrenia with an effect size in the moderate range [279]. CRT is endorsed by the Scottish Intercollegiate Guidelines Network (www.sign.ac.uk/pdf/sign131.pdf). However, as yet, any cognitive improvements do not appear to generalise beyond the specific training task [279].

Avatar therapy is showing considerable promise as a treatment for 'voices', but is at an early stage in terms of definitive evidence [280, 281].

Open dialogue therapy (OD), an intensive talking therapy involving the sufferer and the family, has attracted advocates [282]. However, clinical trials of open-dialogue therapy have been of poor quality with a high risk of bias, precluding any definitive conclusions on efficacy [283, 284].

Other therapies in development include; compassion focused therapy (CFT), acceptance and commitment therapy (ACT), narrative therapy, method of levels therapy (MoL), metacognitive therapy and mindfulness. As yet, the evidence base on which to draw conclusions is less extensive than that for CBT [285].

More generally, some have questioned whether CBT should continue to dominate the other psychotherapies (across psychiatry as a whole) especially given the disappointing results, and if a more diverse approach to therapy provision would be preferable [286]

Compared to treatment as usual, therapy aimed at enhancing medication adherence has been shown to reduce the relapse rate in schizophrenia [122–124] and bipolar disorder [125].

Side effects of antipsychotic treatment

6.1 Weight gain

Weight gain can be a major problem for patients with psychosis. It is very common to encounter patients who have gained 10 kg or more in weight after a relatively short period of treatment with antipsychotics. Not surprisingly, these patients can easily lose faith in the suggestion that maintenance treatment will enhance their lives.

The rate of weight gain is highest after first starting an antipsychotic, and the rate in this initial period is predictive of long-term weight gain [287, 288]. For this reason, it is vital to measure body weight every week during the initiation phase. A nutrition screen at baseline is also recommended (Appendix 3). In time genetic testing may aid prediction [288].

In terms of both the probability and the extent of weight gain, the following ranking of antipsychotic medications is recognised.: [104]

High risk. Clozapine and olanzapine.
Intermediate risk. Quetiapine, chlorpromazine, risperidone, brexpiprazole, iloperidone, cariprazine
Lower risk. Haloperidol, trifluoperazine, amisulpride, aripiprazole, lurasidone, asenapine.

The exact mechanism of antipsychotic induced weight gain is unknown, but increased appetite arising from potent blockade of H_1 and $5HT_{2c}$ receptors on hypothalamic neurons has been implicated [290]. In the hypothalamus, serotonin acts at $5HT_{2c}$ receptors to provide an appetite suppressing signal. Some antipsychotics do not merely block the $5HT_{2c}$ receptor, but act as inverse agonists, switching off any constitutive $5HT_{2c}$ appetite suppression.

6.1.1 Antipsychotics at $5HT_{2c}$ receptors

Clozapine, olanzapine, and risperidone are potent inverse agonists at the $5HT_{2c}$ receptor. Clozapine has a marked preference for $5HT_{2c}$ over D_2 receptors, olanzapine binds equally well to both. This means that at doses in the antipsychotic range $5HT_{2c}$ inverse agonism is unavoidable with clozapine and olanzapine.

Advanced Prescribing in Psychosis, First Edition. Paul Morrison, David M. Taylor and Phillip McGuire.
© 2020 John Wiley & Sons Ltd. Published 2020 by John Wiley & Sons Ltd.

Aripiprazole is a partial agonist at the $5HT_{2c}$ receptor, which may explain why aripiprazole can counteract clozapine and olanzapine induced weight-gain.

6.1.2 The management of weight gain and obesity

Abdominal obesity is a risk factor for type-II diabetes, dyslipidemia and cardiovascular disease.

'Prevention of weight gain is better than cure'. For this reason, physical health monitoring and advice is focused at the early intervention stage. In this phase, patients are generally young and slim, and are more motivated to avoid weight gain than in later life.

A regular assessment of cardiovascular risk factors is required (Appendix 3).

Smoking status, blood-pressure, glucose/Hb1Ac, lipids.
Individual risk factors are additive for adverse cardiovascular outcomes.
Calculate risk using the QRISK2 (http://qrisk.org) if appropriate, see Section 7.3.

Diet and exercise programmes are effective in research settings [291, 292]. Lifestyle modification is the basis of any weight-loss plan for the individual patient [293].

Switch to a weight-neutral antipsychotic (Table 3.7) [294].

Cross-titration to a relatively weight neutral antipsychotic can be effective, but watch for breakthrough insomnia (removal of H_1 antagonism) or breakthrough psychosis.

The following pharmacological add-in strategies have been shown to outperform placebo by approximately ↓2–3 kg on average; Aripiprazole [295], metformin [296], topiramate [297], orlistat [298].

Glucagon-like peptide-1 (GLP-1) receptor agonists (liraglutide, exenatide) outperform placebo by approximately ↓2.4–5 kg on average [299]. A downside is that such agents require subcutaneous administration, although once-weekly formulations have been developed for several molecules in the class.

GLP-1 receptor agonists have been associated with a possible risk of pancreatitis [300]. However, a meta-analysis of randomised controlled trials (RCTs) found no increased risk of pancreatitis [301]. Moreover, a recent clinical trial involving over 9 000 patients found that the incidence of pancreatitis or pancreatic cancer did not differ between GLP-1 receptor agonist versus placebo treated groups [302].

6.2 Type II diabetes

There is evidence of glucose dysregulation from onset of psychosis, even prior to antipsychotic use. Considering diabetic risk from time of diagnosis is therefore recommended [303].

Thresholds for pre-diabetes and type II diabetes are shown in Table 6.1, along with the recommended management.

Weight gain is a risk factor for type-II diabetes, but even in the absence of weight gain, the antipsychotics carry a risk for type II diabetes.

Although the risk of type II diabetes is probably a class effect, which may be mediated in part through D_2 receptors in the pancreas, there are marked differences between individual drugs [304].

Table 6.1 Thresholds for diabetes.

Measure	High risk of type II diabetes	Type II diabetes
Fasting blood glucose (mmol l^{-1})	5.5–6.9	≥7.0
Hb1Ac (mmol mol^{-1})	42–47 (6.0–6.4%)	≥48 (≥6.5%)
Random blood glucose (mmol l^{-1})	—	>11.1
Management	Lifestyle modification. Metformin for prevention.	NICE guidelines NG28 Lifestyle modification. Metformin is 1st line.
Target Hb1Ac (mmol mol^{-1})	<42 (6.0%)	48 (6.5%) if on diet/exercise or metformin 53 (7.0%) if on a sulphonylurea

Clozapine and olanzapine constitute the highest risk for type II diabetes [305]. A possible mechanism is blockade of cholinergic M_3 receptors followed by a downstream adverse impact on insulin signalling. Clozapine has a preference for M_3 over D_2 receptors which means that at doses in the antipsychotic range, M_3 effects are unavoidable. The following ranking is recognised: [104]

Highest risk. clozapine
High risk. olanzapine
Intermediate risk. quetiapine, risperidone, chlorpromazine
Low risk. haloperidol, trifluoperazine
Minimal. amisulpride, aripiprazole, lurasidone.

Although rare, it is important to be alert to symptoms and signs of diabetic ketoacidosis (DKA) which can occur in the absence of weight gain and constitutes a medical emergency requiring hospital admission. Case reports implicate the class, even aripiprazole [306].

- Features of DKA are severe thirst, excessive urination, nausea/vomiting, tiredness, shortness of breath, dehydration, fruit-scented breath (ketones), abdominal pain, confusion, and eventual coma. Biochemistry reveals hyperglycemia, ketonaemia and urinary ketones.

Poorly controlled type II diabetes is a risk factor for microvascular and macrovascular complications. The probability of adverse vascular outcomes increases as risk factors accumulate. Monitoring requirements are shown in appendix 3.

Calculate risk using the QRISK2 (http://qrisk.org) if appropriate, see Section 7.3.

The management of pre-diabetes and type-II diabetes in psychosis services
Switch antipsychotic as per Table 3.7, and re-check Hb1Ac in approximately eight weeks.
Lifestyle modifications encompassing diet, physical exercise and weight management.
Follow NICE guidelines (NG28). www.nice.org.uk/guidance/ng28
Correspond with GP.

CHAPTER 6

Set a target for Hb1Ac. Measure Hb1Ac every three to six months.

The first-line drug treatment of type II diabetes is standard release metformin [307]. Metformin has a low risk of hypoglycemia. Doses are gradually increased over weeks to minimise GI side-effects. If tolerance is an issue, a trial of the modified release preparation can be considered.

Monitor renal function.

eGFR <45 ml min^{-1}/1.73 m^2. Seek specialist advice. Dose reduction?

eGFR <30 ml min^{-1}/1.73 m^2. Stop metformin.

Poor tolerance of metformin *OR* if Hb1Ac rises to >58 mmol mol^{-1} despite metformin:

Liaise with GP.

Refer to consultant-led multidisciplinary diabetes team.

2nd and 3rd line agents include:

DPP-4i (Dipeptidyl peptidase-4 inhibitors).

Pioglitazone.

SU (Sulphonylureas).

SGLT-2i (sodium/glucose co-transporter 2 inhibitors).

Insulin-based treatment.

Diabetes expertise is essential for the 2nd and 3rd line therapies. Co-working between the psychiatric and diabetes teams is ideal.

6.3   Dyslipidemia

Dyslipidemia is a recognised risk factor for cardiovascular disease. Antipsychotics can increase plasma levels of total cholesterol, LDL cholesterol and triglycerides.

Obesity is a cause of dyslipidemia. However, antipsychotic induced dyslipidemia can occur in the absence of weight gain.

Olanzapine and clozapine carry the highest risk, quetiapine and chlorpromazine are intermediate and the others are of low/negligible risk.

6.3.1   The management of dyslipidemia in psychosis services

Switch antipsychotic (Table 3.7) [294]. Re-check lipids in 12 weeks.

Lifestyle modifications encompassing diet, physical exercise and weight management.

Follow NICE guidelines (cg181). www.nice.org.uk/guidance/cg181

Calculate risk using the QRISK2 (http://qrisk.org).

except if: pre-existing cardiovascular disease, type-I diabetes, renal disease, familial hypercholesterolemia

Risk assessment tools such as the QRISK2 underestimate cardiovascular risk in patients taking antipsychotics.

Correspond with GP.

NICE recommends that if the 10-year risk of developing cardiovascular disease ≥10%, offer atorvastatin 20 mg for primary prevention.

Carry out a full lipid profile at baseline: Total cholesterol, high density lipoprotein (HDL) cholesterol, LDL cholesterol, and triglycerides. *NICE recommends that a fasting sample is not needed.*

Secondary causes of dyslipidemia: poorly controlled diabetes, excess alcohol, liver disease, nephrotic syndrome.

Seek expert opinion if:

Total cholesterol >7.5 mmol l^{-1} + family history of premature coronary heart disease. Familial hypercholesterolemia?

- Total cholesterol >9.0 mmol l^{-1} or non-HDL cholesterol >7.5 mmol l^{-1}.
- Triglyceride concentration >10 mmol l^{-1} on two consecutive tests, between 5 and 14 days apart, the second of which is under fasting conditions.
- Triglyceride concentration >4.5 mmol $^{-1}$ + non-HDL cholesterol >7.5 mmol l^{-1}.
- Urgent expert opinion if:
- Triglyceride concentration >20 mmol l^{-1} *not accounted for by excess alcohol or poor diabetic control.*

The decision to begin a statin for primary prevention will usually be taken in liaison with the patient's GP. In addition to a full lipid profile, LFTs, renal function, thyroid function tests are checked at baseline.

6.4   Motor side effects

Many antipsychotic drugs can cause motor side effects, as a consequence of excessive dopamine D$_2$ receptor blockade in the basal ganglia.

As part of normal physiology within the basal ganglia, dopamine is essential for the selection, implementation and switching of psychomotor programmes [308].

In addition, very precise dopamine signals are involved in embedding new psychomotor programmes as learned habits within the basal ganglia network [308, 309].

Disruption of dopamine signalling in the basal ganglia can give rise to dystonia, Parkinsonism, akathisia and tardive dyskinesia (TD), the latter arising from abnormal plasticity within the network. The features and management of these extra-pyramidal side effects (EPSEs) are shown in Table 6.2.

Drugs which have high affinity for the dopamine D$_2$ receptor carry a significant risk for EPSEs (Table 3.1).

The 1st generation ('typical') antipsychotics are regarded as high risk but dose is a critical factor. By the mid-1990s, PET and SPECT imaging demonstrated that many antipsychotics have a narrow therapeutic window in the basal ganglia. It became clear that sufficient D$_2$ blockade is necessary for an antipsychotic effect, but there is a narrow margin before EPSEs begin to emerge.

A previous era had seen a fashion for high-dose prescribing, indeed the upper dose limit of many first-generation drugs is high and somewhat arbitrary. By the mid-1990s, it was clear that increasing the dose above the therapeutic window made Parkinsonian side effects more likely but did not confer any additional antipsychotic effect [310].

Table 6.2 Extra-pyramidal side effects.

	Dystonia	Parkinsonism	Akathisia	Tardive dyskinesia
Features	Intense muscle spasm. *Commonly eye muscles, neck, tongue.*	Difficulty initiating movement. *Commonly muscles of facial expression.* Tremor (3–5 Hz). Muscle rigidity. Salivary drooling. Slowed thinking.	Motor restlessness and subjective inner tension. *Commonly limb muscles.* *Relationship with suicidal thoughts/acts.*	Abnormal involuntary movements mainly of the tongue and mouth. May be irreversible. Early akathisia and Parkinsonism is a risk factor for TD.
Timing *Following initiation or dose increase.*	Within hours.	Within days to months.	Within days.	Months to years.
Anti-cholinergics?	Highly effective	Effective	Unhelpful	Unhelpful, can worsen.
Management	IM anticholinergics Thereafter switch antipsychotic.	Distinguish from depression and negative symptoms. ↓ dose or switch antipsychotic. Oral anticholinergic *Short-term only.*	Concurrent SSRI? SSRIs can cause akathisia. SSRIs can inhibit antipsychotic metabolism (Appendix 1) dose or switch antipsychotic. Add-in? Benzodiazepine *Short-term only.* Propanolol *Risk in overdose* *Avoid in asthma* Mirtazapine *Weight-gain & sedation.*	Switch antipsychotic Quetiapine? Clozapine? Tetrabenazine Deutetrabenazine Valbenazine *Deplete nerve varicosities of monoamines. Also have antipsychotic properties but monitor for depression & sedation.* Pyridoxine (Vit. B6) Ginkgo biloba *Anti-platelet effect. Caution in patients using anticoagulants/antiplatelet agents.* Clonazepam *Drowsiness*

Drugs which have high affinity for muscarinic acetylcholine receptors in the basal
ganglia have a reduced propensity for EPSEs. This is the case for thioridazine (now
discontinued) and olanzapine.

It was believed that antagonism of serotonin $5HT_{2a}$ receptors protected against EPSEs,
but many of the first-generation drugs have high affinity for $5HT_{2a}$ receptors. Also
the addition of a pure $5HT_{2a}$ antagonist to a potent D_2 regime has no discernible
effect on EPSEs.

Quetiapine and clozapine have low affinity for the dopamine D_2 receptor, and
relatively higher affinity for muscarinic acetylcholine receptors. The risk of EPSEs are
negligible to the extent that clozapine (but probably not quetiapine) is a treatment
option in psychosis arising in the context of idiopathic Parkinson's disease [311]. A new
agent, pimavanserin, an inverse agonist at $5HT_{2A}$ and $5HT_{2C}$ receptors, may have efficacy for psychosis occurring in Parkinson's disease [312, 313], although there has been
some controversy [314].

Risperidone, amisulpride, ziprasidone, and asenapine can cause EPSEs.

Aripiprazole, cariprazine, and lurasidone are associated with akathisia.

6.4.1 Tardive dyskinesia

Amongst the EPSEs, tardive dyskinesa (TD) is probably the most feared because it can
be irreversible and markedly disfiguring.

Early EPSEs are a risk factor for TD. If EPSEs arise, basal ganglia D_2 blockade is
excessive, and doses need adjusted.

6.4.2 First versus second generation

It was assumed that the second generation ('atypical') antipsychotics would be devoid
of the propensity to cause TD, but it has become clear that the risk from second-generation drugs, as a group, is only modestly lower (*approx. 0.7*) than the first-generation
drugs [315].

It probably makes more sense, however, to consider each drug on its own merit and
abandon the typical v atypical distinction [316]. For example, quetiapine and clozapine carry a negligible risk of TD, and represent viable switches in established TD.
Furthermore, clozapine can improve established TD [317, 318].

6.5 Hyperprolactinemia

Prolactin is a pituitary hormone whose best known role is the stimulation of breast
tissue to grow and produce milk after childbirth. In normal physiology, a set of
dopamine neurons in the hypothalamus keep prolactin under inhibitory control.
Antipsychotic drugs can block this inhibitory signal (D_2 receptor effect) causing elevated
prolactin in the bloodstream (hyperprolactinemia) [84].

Hyperprolactinemia: Prolactin levels $>424\,\mathrm{mIUl^{-1}}$ ($20\,\mathrm{\mu gl^{-1}}$) in men; $>530\,\mathrm{mIUl^{-1}}$
($25\,\mathrm{\mu gl^{-1}}$) in women.

The consequences of high prolactin include the following:

Decreased libido.
Irregular periods or cessation of periods.
Growth of breast tissue.
Lactation.
Longer term: bone thinning. Risk of fractures [319].

Recommendations from the British Association of Psychopharmacology (BAP) are to avoid hyperprolactinemia in:

Patients who have not reached peak bone mass (age <25 years).
Women wishing to become pregnant.
Patients with osteoporosis.
Patients with a previous history of breast cancer.

In the context of antipsychotic prescribing, prolactin levels should be checked at baseline and at three-months after a dose increase.In the atypical class, amisulpride, paliperidone, and risperidone are particularly associated with hyperprolactinemia.

Amisulpride has a propensity for hyperprolactinemia because it penetrates the brain poorly, but the concomitant high-bloodstream concentrations have free access to the pituitary gland.

6.5.1   The management of hyperprolactinemia

If pituitary symptoms pre-medication OR prolactin levels $>2500 \, mIU l^{-1}$ ($118 \, \mu g l^{-1}$) seek endocrinology opinion to exclude adenoma.
The following options are available:

Switch antipsychotic (See Table 3.4)
Add in aripiprazole.
Aripiprazole is a high-affinity D_2 partial agonist which generally out-competes other anti-psychotics at the D_2 receptor, with the exception of amisulpride. By eight weeks, aripiprazole can normalise the prolactin level in over 95% of patients [320, 321].
No change if asymptomatic hyperprolactinemia and not in a high-risk group.
Rather than treating a blood result in isolation, it is important to see the whole patient and the previous history. Many patients are stable, well, have no physical symptoms of hyperprolactinemia and are not in an at-risk group with respect to bone density.
Clinical judgement is needed to decide if switching to another antipsychotic is likely to confer more benefit than risk. There is time to obtain an endocrinology opinion, as it will take several months for prolactin levels to normalise.

6.6   Sexual side effects

Sexual side effects are often overlooked and not asked about. Psychotropic medication can impact upon sexual desire, arousal, and orgasm. Sexual dysfunction occurs in approximately 50% of patients [61].

Sexual side effects cannot be explained entirely by effects on prolactin. Serotonin, noradrenaline, dopamine, nitric oxide, and acetylcholine are involved in the central and/or peripheral regulation of sexual responses [322–324]. For example, antipsychotic drugs block dopamine signals in the medial pre-optic nucleus, an important hub in the control of sexual behaviour [325].

Antipsychotics can impact upon desire, arousal and orgasm.
  The propensity for sexual side effects is as follows (highest to lowest): [326]
  risperidone > haloperidol > olanzapine > quetiapine > aripiprazole

6.6.1 Management

Assess for hyperprolactinemia (Section 6.5)
  On selective serotonin reuptake inhibitor (SSRI)? SSRIs commonly delay orgasm (*paroxetine most*) [327].
  Consider a switch of antipsychotic.
  Phosphodiesterase type 5 (PDE5) inhibitors such as sildenafil are effective for impaired sexual arousal in men and women [328, 329].

6.7 Prolonged QTc

Several antipsychotics can block a voltage sensitive K+ channel on heart muscle cells called the hERG channel (*human-ether-a-go-go-related gene*). The hERG channel is fairly promiscuous for a range of drugs because of a large binding pocket in the pore channel. In drug development, the hERG channel is an important *anti*-target [330].

In normal physiology, opening of the hERG channel helps to bring the heart muscle back to resting potential following brief electrical excitation. Impaired functioning of hERG can delay cardiac repolarisation, which manifests as a prolonged QT interval on the ECG [331].

Loss of function mutations in hERG account for about one-third of inherited long QT syndromes [332]. Other genetic causes of long QT arise from mutations in other types of K+ channel, Na+ channels, Ca^2 channels, or in auxiliary proteins which provide a scaffold for the channels [333].

The prevalence of genetic long QT syndromes is ~1 in 2000.
Warning features are faints during exercise and a family history of sudden cardiac death before 40.

6.7.1 Calculating the QTc

The QT interval is the total time period for ventricular depolarisation + ventricular repolarisation. It is calculated from the start of the Q-wave to the end of the T-wave [334]. QT intervals vary significantly among ECG leads [335]. Most normal reference ranges are based upon measurements from lead II [336].

The QT interval depends on the heart rate; as heart rate increases QT decreases. The QT is corrected for heart rate yielding the QTc. At 60 bpm QT = QTc. There are various

CHAPTER 6

methods for calculating the QTc of which Bazett's formula is the most widely known (*QTc = the QT interval in milliseconds/the square root of the heart rate in seconds*) [334].

A limitation of Bazett's formula is that it is inaccurate at heart rate extremes, for example producing overlong QTc values at faster heart rates (particularly >85 bpm) [337]. There are alternatives for faster rates e.g. Fredericia, although none are perfect [338].

6.7.2   QTc thresholds

Precise figures vary but a QTc of up to 440 ms in men and 470 ms in women is regarded as normal [334].

QTc values >500 ms increase the risk of torsades de pointes. The risk is exponential, 1% at 500 ms, 50% at 600 ms. [334]

6.7.3   Torsades de points

Long QTc may be asymptomatic, but is a risk factor for abnormal excitation in heart muscle and torsades de pointes. Torsades de pointes usually manifests as faints and seizures. Most episodes revert to spontaneous sinus rhythm, but some persist and progress to ventricular fibrillation and sudden cardiac death.

Most cases of drug-associated torsades de pointes occur in patients with multiple risk factors: older patients; bradycardia, previous MI, heart failure; renal failure; electrolyte abnormality, low K^+, or Mg^{2+}.

Low K^+ or Mg^{2+} can be caused by anorexia nervosa, malnourishment, chronic alcoholism, vomiting, diarrhoea, or K^+ depleting diuretics.

An updated list of drugs which can cause prolonged QTc is at www.crediblemeds.org. The following are recognised:

Antiarrhythmics: amiodarone, sotalol, disopyramide, quinidine, procainamide
Macrolide antibiotics: azithromycin, clarithromycin, erythromycin
Antifungals: ketoconazole, fluconazole
Antivirals: nelfinavir
Antimalarials: chloroquine, mefloquine
Methadone
Certain antihistamines terfenadine
Tricyclics imipramine, amitriptyline, nortriptyline, desipramine, dosulepin
Citalopram >40 mg d^{-1}.

6.7.4   Antipsychotics and QTc prolongation

Higher risk (↑ >20 ms) agents are thioridazine, sertindole, pimozide, ziprasidone, and IV haloperidol [176].

The affinity of thioridazine, sertindole and pimozide for the hERG channel is close to their affinity for the dopamine D_2 receptor, which means that blockade of hERG is likely with these agents in the antipsychotic dose range. Thioridazine was withdrawn because of concern over arrhythmia and sudden cardiac death, whereas sertindole and pimozide come with black box warnings and are now rarely prescribed [176]. IV haloperidol carries a substantial risk of long QT and torsades de pointes [339].

For the other commonly prescribed antipsychotics, QTc usually only becomes a concern in cases of overdose, impaired drug metabolism, if there are other risk factors present or when antipsychotics are used in combination with other drugs which can prolong the QTc [176].

Intermediate risk (↑ 7–15 ms): Quetiapine, chlorpromazine
Low risk (↑ 3–10 ms): Clozapine, olanzapine, risperidone, amisulpride haloperidol, flu-
  phenazine, flupentixol, aripiprazole, paliperidone, iloperidone, asenapine
No effect on QTc: lurasidone, brexpiprazole, cariprazine
Unknown: zuclopenthixol, trifluoperazine.

6.7.5 Management

QTc values >500 ms.
Review risk-factors.
Review medications. Doses. Combinations. Interactions.
Prompt discussion with cardiologist. Consider transthoracic echo, 24-hour tape.
Switch to an antipsychotic with lower risk of prolonged QTc.
Consider

'Borderline' QTc <500 ms.
Review risk-factors.
Review medications. Doses. Combinations. Interactions.
Discuss with cardiologist.
Consider switching to an antipsychotic with lower risk of prolonged QTc.
Liaise with cardiologist in regard to the utility of an implantable cardioverter-defibrillator
  (ICD) if the severity of the psychiatric condition warrants clozapine continuation.

6.8 Neuroleptic malignant syndrome

Neuroleptic malignant syndrome (NMS) is a rare but major side effect of all antipsychotic medications. High-potency D_2 drugs carry the highest risk, especially if there are rapid dose increases or reductions [104].

Patients with Lewy-body dementia are at high risk because of sensitivity to antipsychotics. Other drugs associated with NMS include: lithium, tricyclic antidepressants, reserpine, and tetrabenazine or the rapid withdrawal of L-DOPA.

The mortality from NMS has dropped because of better recognition and robust early treatment.
  Clinical features are:

muscle cramps, rigidity
fever, sweating

CHAPTER 6

autonomic instability, e.g. fluctuating blood pressure
fluctuating mental state; confusion, agitation, coma
metabolic acidosis

Laboratory features are:

↑ creatine kinase (CK)
↑ white cell count
Altered LFTs.

6.8.1 Management

NMS is a medical emergency, treatment can be lifesaving:
(i). Stop antipsychotic. (ii). Monitor temp, pulse and BP. (iii). Treat hyperthermia robustly (cooling blankets/ice packs). (iv). Discuss transfer to medical unit with physicians. (v). Consider prescribing a benzodiazepine, IM lorazepam.

In the medical unit:
(i). Rehydrate (ii). Ventilation if required (iii). Pharmacological options: bromocriptine + dantrolene for NMS, benzodiazepines for sedation.

Restarting antipsychotics

Let NMS resolve fully.
Avoid high potency D_2 drugs and all depots.
Use low D_2 potency drug, quetiapine or clozapine.
Low dose, titrate slowly.
Close monitoring of physical and biochemical markers.

Chapter 7

Services: pathway specific care

7.1 Background

By the mid-1980s, a series of ground breaking studies from the USA had shown that acute psychotic crises could be treated effectively and safely at home, sparing patients an admission to hospital [340]. Since then, community based multidisciplinary teams have proliferated. In the UK, community teams solely focused on psychosis became commonplace. Psychosis services were then split into those for first-episode patients and those for more chronic patients, in the hope that an enhanced package of treatment as early as possible in the first episode might possibly curtail a decline into chronic schizophrenia. A further specialisation saw the emergence of services in the USA, Australia and the UK targeting the high-risk stage, with the goal of preventing psychosis from establishing any roots at all in the developing psyche.

Sub-specialisation concentrates multidisciplinary expertise on a particular stage or aspect of psychosis. The downside can be that there is less continuity of care, an expansion of management/bureaucracy, and bottlenecks in the transfer of patients from one service to another within a trust [341].

In the South London & Maudsley NHS trust, the clinical services for psychosis are subdivided according to the stage of the disorder being managed. Thus, there are different teams for early intervention (EI), promoting recovery, patients who require acute treatment in hospital, and patients in whom conventional treatment is ineffective (http://www.slam.nhs.uk/about-us/clinical-academic-groups/psychosis). Below we describe how prescribing varies depending on the stage of psychosis.

7.2 The at-risk-mental-state

Specialist clinics for the at-risk-mental state for psychosis have emerged over the last two decades [342]. In the South London & Maudsley Trust (SLAM) the at-risk clinic is known as OASIS (Outreach & support in South London). The diagnosis of the

Advanced Prescribing in Psychosis, First Edition. Paul Morrison, David M. Taylor and Phillip McGuire.
© 2020 John Wiley & Sons Ltd. Published 2020 by John Wiley & Sons Ltd.

at-risk-mental state is based on specific clinical criteria [343]. Three subtypes have been defined:

1. Those who experience a psychotic episode (<1-week duration) which resolves without treatment; termed a brief limited intermittent psychosis (BLIP).
2. Those with sub-threshold ('attenuated') positive symptoms.
3. Those with a family history of a psychotic disorder in a first-degree relative + psychosocial decline over at least one year.
4. Of these three subtypes, BLIPs carry the highest risk for transition to a psychotic illness. BLIPs are synonymous with an acute transient psychotic disorder [8, 344].

In the at-risk-mental state, there is a high prevalence of comorbidity, particularly depression and anxiety [345, 346].

The risk of transition to a full blown psychotic disorder over three years varies from centre to centre, depending on the nature of the population ascertained at each site, from 10% to 30%. If an individual at high risk is going to develop psychosis, it will usually occur within two to three years of clinical presentation [347, 348].

Although there have been reports that psychological interventions might decrease the rate of transition to psychosis [349–352], the largest and most rigorous study involving 288 participants found that cognitive behavioural therapy (CBT) did not reduce the transition to psychosis [265].

A recent network analysis found that there is no evidence that any specific intervention, including CBT, prevents transition to psychosis [266]

Nevertheless, despite the lack of an evidence base CBT has been recommended as the treatment of choice in the NICE guidelines (www.nice.org.uk/guidance/CG178).

Antipsychotic medications are not recommended in this population because of a high sensitivity to adverse effects and concerns about stigmatisation [343].

It is recommended that care should be provided for at least two years, which approximately reflects the period of maximal risk of transition to psychosis [343].

7.3 Early intervention services

Early intervention (EI) services utilise multidisciplinary expertise and aim to improve the long-term outcome of patients suffering the early stages of psychosis. Medication of psychotic symptoms occurs alongside an intensive treatment package aimed at re-integration and recovery which can include individual psychology, family work, group work and vocational support, in addition to care coordinator input.

Patients who experience delays of over one or more year in accessing antipsychotic medication have more persistent positive and negative symptoms, and are more likely to show functional decline and cognitive impairment [93, 353–355].

There is research evidence that, compared to standard care, EI can improve clinical outcomes, in the first few years [356–358] with no apparent increase of financial cost [359]. It is less clear if the clinical benefits are sustained in the longer term, although this may require that specialised care is provided for longer than the initial one to two years that is typically provided [360, 361].

7.4   Acute services

Acute services in SLAM are organised around the home treatment team (HTT). The HTT allows people in the midst of a psychotic crisis to be treated safely at home. The HTT also acts as a gatekeeper to hospital admission [362].

The most common cause of relapse is discontinuation of medication. HTT staff are skilled in supporting patients and their families, supervising medication, titrating doses, monitoring progress, and judging risk. Short-term benzodiazepines, z-drugs and sedative antihistamines can be useful adjuncts in a crisis. Oro-dispersible antipsychotic medication can also be helpful.

Some patients cannot be treated at home and need hospital admission. There are various reasons such as refusal to work with the HTT or excessive risk. In some cases, compulsory detention under the mental health act is necessary.

With fewer and fewer beds, there is a risk that the wards become short-stay holding areas for the most acutely agitated and high-risk patients and that the function of the psychiatric hospital as place of sanctuary and respite becomes increasingly historical [363].

Upon discharge from hospital, many patients benefit from a period under the care of the HTT before going back to the parent community team [364]. This can be helpful for ensuring that clinical improvements are sustained, when patients return to their former environments and the stresses therein.

7.5   Continuing care services: promoting recovery

Current practice in SLAM is that patients remain with the early intervention team for up to three years [365]. Thereafter, a proportion of patients will be referred to the Promoting Recovery service. Generally, this service will provide care for patients with an established functional psychiatric syndrome, usually schizophrenia, schizoaffective or bipolar disorder.

There has been a move to re-orientate mental health services towards promoting wellbeing rather than treating illness, using positive psychology and individual narratives of recovery [366, 367]. The hope is that the provision of resources to enhance wellbeing will enable the individual to manage their own healthcare [368, 369].

The prognosis for schizophrenia is far better than was believed in the past [369, 370]. Over the long-term only about 10–15% of patients will show a severely disabled picture, but the majority will make a significant recovery, and about 20% will recover fully. Even negative symptoms, a core component of schizophrenia, show a recovery over time [371].

A package of multidisciplinary care concentrates the expertise of social workers, occupational therapists, psychologists, nurses and psychiatrists on a patient's re-integration and recovered quality of life.

Some patients need a package of rehabilitative care to be able to begin their recovery, Rehabilitative care can be delivered in designated wards or in the community.

For users of rehabilitation services, positive outcomes (*community discharge* or a less *supported community placement*) are predicted by adherence to medication [372].

As time goes by, psychotic symptoms in schizophrenia usually become less intense and may burn out altogether. Many patients learn to no longer feel overwhelmed or threatened by their positive symptoms, and insight can develop.

A desired outcome of community mental health teams (CMHTs) is the return of patients to primary care. However, 58% of patients will be re-referred in the first year, with 60% of those in crisis [373].

Chapter 8

Measuring outcomes

Two main types of outcome are assessed in healthcare systems; those which measure direct clinical outcomes for patients and those which measure the process of healthcare delivery itself. An example of the former, as pertains to major mental illness, is a reduction in relapse rates and re-admission. Examples of the latter might be whether a caseload '*achieves*' an arbitrarily-set target of ICD10 diagnoses, blood-tests, offers of cognitive behavioural therapy (CBT), waiting-times and so forth.

8.1   Value-based healthcare

Value-based healthcare (VBH) is emerging as a way of analysing outcomes and cost, whereby clinical gains of direct clinical relevance for patients are given priority over measures of the healthcare delivery process itself.

To calculate value, clinical gains are measured versus cost. Clinical gains are denoted by the numerator whereas the total cost of the treatment (including all management/bureaucratic overheads) is denoted by the denominator [374].

VBH can be highly informative [375]. For example, a spreadsheet approach may show that a particular drug is considerably more expensive than alternatives, and an impulsive decision may be made to limit prescribing of the expensive drug. However, if additional variables are incorporated, the conclusion can alter. For instance, the more expensive drug may result in fewer hospital re-admissions, resource savings and increased value [376].

The use of standard rating scales to quantify clinical gains are rare, even in major research-orientated psychiatric trusts. Rating scales, of course, do not capture the nuances of improvement, but they generate a number which can be used to track change.

A large population of patients combined with a database of their searchable electronic records is ideal for addressing a whole host of clinical unknowns and for optimising value.

Advanced Prescribing in Psychosis, First Edition. Paul Morrison, David M. Taylor and Phillip McGuire.
© 2020 John Wiley & Sons Ltd. Published 2020 by John Wiley & Sons Ltd.

Table 8.1 Outcome rating scales.

Scale	Domain	Characteristics	Download
CGI, *Clinical Global Impression*	A global rating of severity and response to treatment.	Extensive use in research Quick & easy to use Three items: severity, global improvement and efficacy	www.psywellness.com.sg/docs/CGI.pdf
GAF, *Global assessment of functioning scale*	A global rating of psychological, occupational and social functioning.	Extensive use in research Quick & easy to use One item	https://msu.edu/course/sw/840/stocks/pack/axisv.pdf
PANSS, *Positive & negative syndrome scale*	The symptoms and signs of schizophrenia.	Extensive use in research Seven positive items Seven negative items 16 general items Rating of positive items is quick and easy	http://www.emotionalwellbeing.southcentral.nhs.uk/resources/doc_download/62-panss-positive-and-negative-syndrome-scale-pdf-document
GASS, *Glasgow antipsychotic side-effect scale*	Rates the common side effects of antipsychotics.	Quick & easy to use. Patient completed questionnaire 20 items	https://mentalhealthpartnerships.com/resource/glasgow-antipsychotic-side-effect-scale/

Scales such as the clinical global impression (CGI) and global assessment of functioning (GAF) are very easy to use and capture global change, as well as being valid research instruments acceptable for publication. Other scales (Table 6.2) which measure symptoms and side effects are shown in Table 8.1. The advantage of the CGI and GAF is that they *apply* numbers to the intuitive holistic sense (Gestalt) of whether a patient is improving, or not.

8.2   Evidence-based healthcare management (EBMGT)

The management of healthcare is at last beginning to adopt mathematical and engineering principles. There is an awareness that decisionmaking in complex systems requires mathematical thinking allied with powerful computer modelling [377, 378].

Complex systems are made up of many components. A decision which impacts upon one component in a healthcare system may affect other components, and indeed the whole system, in a way which was not predicted at the outset [378–380]. Quite often a decision aimed at conserving resource, can actually end up leaking resources as unforeseen consequences emerge, necessitating another cycle of rash decision making [381].

Managers/leaders can perform computer based-simulations rather than implementing change in the absence of data. Discrete event simulation (DES) is one such method.

It is far less costly, and hazardous, to perform and learn from DES, than to implement change directly into the healthcare system.

The next generation of managers/leaders need to be equipped with the prerequisite mathematical skills to ensure that maximum resource is delivered to a maximum number of patients, and that the cost of management/bureaucracy is itself minimised.

Mathematical modelling of complex systems, such as healthcare, can provide insight into how change in one component affects other parts of the system [382]. With a deeper analysis of the system, decisions can be taken with less uncertainty over downstream consequences [341].

An important aspect is the feedback loop, which analyses the consequences of a decision. This brings decisionmaking under the gaze of the scientific method, and constitutes evidence-based management *(EBMgt)* [378].

A healthcare delivery service, including all managerial/bureaucratic components is recognised as a complex *adaptive* system [383, 384]. Adaption signifies that the system learns from feedback and moves over-time, ever closer towards an optimal configuration. Due to the sheer number of variables, mathematical modelling is the only feasible way for guiding a complex system towards an optimal configuration [385].

Pharmacokinetics of selected psychotropics

Drug	Time to peak plasma concentration t_{max}	Metabolism	Active metabolite	Half-life $t_{1/2}$
Aripiprazole	Oral: 3–5 h Fast-acting IM: 1–3 h	CYP2D6 CYP3A4	Dehydro-aripiprazole	Oral aripiprazole: 75 h

Poor CYP2D6 or CYP3A4 metabolisers.
   Reduce dose by 25–50% and review.

Concomitant inhibition of CYP3A4 OR CYP2D6.
   Reduce oral aripiprazole by 50%.

Concomitant inhibition of CYP3A4 AND CYP2D6.
   Reduce oral aripiprazole by 75%.

Concomitant induction of CYP3A4
   Increase oral aripiprazole and review.

Drug	Time to peak plasma concentration t_{max}	Metabolism	Active metabolite	Half-life $t_{1/2}$
Amisulpride	3–4 h	Renal excretion mostly as unchanged drug	—	12 h

Caution in renal impairment.
   Creatinine clearance (CC) 30–60 ml min⁻¹: reduce dose by 50%.
   CC 10–30 ml min⁻¹: reduce dose by two-thirds.
   Concomitant lithium increases plasma amisulpride concentrations.

Drug	Time to peak plasma concentration t_{max}	Metabolism	Active metabolite	Half-life $t_{1/2}$
Quetiapine	1.5 h	CYP3A4	norquetiapine	6–7 h

Caution in renal or hepatic impairment.
   Caution with concomitant inhibitors of CYP3A4.
   Concomitant induction of CYP3A4: Higher doses of quetiapine may be necessary.
   Norquetiapine is a noradrenaline re-uptake inhibitor.

Advanced Prescribing in Psychosis, First Edition. Paul Morrison, David M. Taylor and Phillip McGuire.
© 2020 John Wiley & Sons Ltd. Published 2020 by John Wiley & Sons Ltd.

Drug	Time to peak plasma concentration t_{max}	Metabolism	Active metabolite	Half-life $t_{\frac{1}{2}}$
Risperidone	Oral: 1–2 h	CYP2D6	9-hydroxy-risperidone	Oral risperidone (& 9-hydroxyrisperidone): 24h

Initial and consecutive doses should be halved in patients with renal or hepatic impairment.
Risperidone+9-hydroxyrisperidone constitute the active antipsychotic fraction.

Drug	Time to peak plasma concentration t_{max}	Metabolism	Active metabolite	Half-life $t_{\frac{1}{2}}$
Olanzapine	Oral: 5–8 h Fast-acting IM: 15–45 min	CYP1A2 CYP2D6 CYP3A4	—	30–38 h

Reduce starting dose in hepatic impairment.
Fluvoxamine significantly inhibits the metabolism of olanzapine.
The clearance of olanzapine is increased by tobacco smoking.
Neutropenia is more common when olanzapine is given with valproate.
There is an increased incidence of weight gain when olanzapine is given with lithium or valproate.
Fast-acting IM olanzapine: Avoid administration of IM olanzapine+parenteral benzodiazepines within 2 hours, because of potential for excessive sedation and cardiorespiratory depression.

Clozapine	2.5 h	CYP1A2 CYP2D6??	norclozapine	12 h

Target clozapine plasma concentrations >0.35–0.5 mg l^{-1} (Trough).
Caution in renal or hepatic impairment.
Dose titration under medical supervision due to risk of orthostatic hypotension, tachycardia.
Mandatory white blood cell and differential blood counts.
Risk of seizures in a plasma-level dependent manner.
Should not be used alongside drugs with a high risk of bone marrow suppression (e.g. carbamazepine)
Long-acting depots carry a risk of neutropenia, and cannot be withdrawn quickly, and hence should not be used alongside clozapine.
Fluvoxamine (×10), fluoxetine (×2), and paroxetine (×2) increase plasma clozapine concentrations.
Risperidone increases plasma clozapine concentrations.
Tobacco smoke decreases plasma clozapine concentrations.

Lurasidone	1–3 h	CYP3A4	Y	20–40 h

Plasma concentrations are increased by 2–3 times when taken with food v fasting.
Caution in renal or hepatic impairment.

Haloperidol	Oral: 2–6 h Fast-acting IM: 20–30 min	CYP3A4 CYP2D6	—	14–37 h

Contraindicated with other drugs which prolong QTc and K$^+$ depleting diuretics.
Baseline ECG recommended, especially in elderly or positive personal or family history of CVS disease or CVS symptoms/signs.
Caution in hepatic impairment.
Concomitant CYP3A4 or CYPD26 inhibitors can increase haloperidol concentrations including: buspirone, venlafaxine, alprazolam, fluvoxamine, fluoxetine, sertraline, paroxetine, and promethazine.
Concomitant carbamazepine can reduce haloperidol concentrations.
Haloperidol can increase TCA concentrations.
Caution with lithium. Acute confusion+motor symptoms.

Drug	Time to peak plasma concentration t_{max}	Metabolism	Active metabolite	Half-life $t_{1/2}$
Chlorpromazine	Oral 1–4 h	CYP2D6 CYP1A2	—	23–37 h

Contraindicated in renal and hepatic failure, active liver disease, epilepsy, cardiac failure, prostate hypertrophy, pheochromocytoma, myasthenia gravis, and narrow angle glaucoma.
Potentiates the effect of other CNS depressants, anti-hypertensives (esp. α_1 antagonists, ACE inhibitors, Ca^{2+} channel blockers), and anti-muscarinics.
Avoid other drugs which prolong QTc and K^+ depleting diuretics.
High-dose chlorpromazine reduces the response to hypoglycemic agents, the dose of which may need adjustment.
Concomitant CYP1A2 or CYPD26 inhibitors can increase chlorpromazine concentrations.

Drug	Time to peak plasma concentration t_{max}	Metabolism	Active metabolite	Half-life $t_{1/2}$
Flupentixol	Oral 3–6 h	?	—	19–36 h

Caution in renal or hepatic impairment.
Avoid in agitated or excitable patients, may exacerbate these features.
Avoid other drugs which prolong QTc and K^+ depleting diuretics.

Drug	Time to peak plasma concentration t_{max}	Metabolism	Active metabolite	Half-life $t_{1/2}$
Zuclopenthixol	Oral 3–6 h Short-acting IM clopixol acuphase: 36 h	CYP3A4 CYP2D6	—	~20 h

Caution in hepatic impairment.
In renal failure, reduce dose by 50%

Drug	Time to peak plasma concentration t_{max}	Metabolism	Active metabolite	Half-life $t_{1/2}$
Brexpiprazole	Oral 4 h 10–12 d to reach steady state	CYP3A4 CYP2D6	—	91 h

Dose adjustment in renal or hepatic impairment.
In moderate to severe renal or hepatic impairment, do not exceed $2\,mg\,d^{-1}$ in depression and $3\,mg\,d^{-1}$ in schizophrenia.
Poor CYP2D6 metabolisers: reduce dose by 50%.
Poor CYP2D6 metabolisers AND strong CYP3A4 inhibitor: reduce brexpiprazole dose to 25%.
Strong CYP3A4 OR CYP2D6 inhibitors: reduce dose by 50%.
Strong CYP3A4 AND CYP2D6 inhibitors: reduce dose by 50%.
Strong CYP3A4 inducers: Double usual brexpiprazole dose over 1–2 weeks.

Drug	Time to peak plasma concentration t_{max}	Metabolism	Active metabolite	Half-life $t_{1/2}$
Asenapine	Sub-lingual 1 h	CYP1A2	—	24 h

Caution in hepatic impairment.
Contraindicated in severe hepatic impairment.
Fluvoxamine increases plasma concentrations of asenapine. Caution.
Asenapine is a weak inhibitor of CYP2D6. Increases paroxetine concentrations in plasma ×2.

Drug	Time to peak plasma concentration t_{max}	Metabolism	Active metabolite	Half-life $t_{1/2}$
Cariprazine	3–6 h	CYP3A4 CYP2D6	DCAR DDCAR	cariprazine 24–48 h DDCAR 1–3 wk

Steady state at; 1–2 weeks for cariprazine & DCAR, but 4–8 weeks and even up to 12 weeks for DDCAR.
At 12-weeks plasma concentrations of DDCAR are 400% greater than cariprazine.
Strong CYP3A4 inhibitors: reduce dose by 50%.
Strong CYP3A4 inducers: Manufacturer recommends to avoid using strong CYP3A4 inducers with cariprazine.

Drug	Time to peak plasma concentration t_{max}	Metabolism	Active metabolite	Half-life $t_{1/2}$
Iloperidone	2–4 h	CYP3A4 CYP2D6	+	18 h

Drug	Time to peak plasma concentration t_{max}	Metabolism	Active metabolite	Half-life $t_{1/2}$
	Dose adjustment in moderate hepatic impairment. Poor CYP2D6 metabolisers: reduce dose by 50%. Strong CYP3A4 AND/OR CYP2D6 inhibitors: reduce dose by 50%.			
Ziprasidone	4–5 h	CYP3A4		Single dose 4–5 h Repeat doses 9–10 h
	Absorption enhanced by food. Avoid other drugs which prolong QTc and K^+ depleting diuretics.			
Lithium carbonate (prolonged release)	2 h	Renal excretion	—	18–36 h
	Contraindicated in patients with severe renal insufficiency. Mild/moderate renal insufficiency: monitor Li^+ plasma levels closely. ■ Toxicity: plasma levels of 1.5 mmol l^{-1}. ■ NSAIDs, ACE inhibitors, diuretics, steroids, tetracyclines can ↑ Li^+ plasma levels. ■ Avoid dehydration. Caution with antipsychotics (especially higher dose haloperidol). Acute confusion + motor symptoms. Caution with serotonergic antidepressants. Serotonin syndrome. Caution with Ca^{2+} channel antagonists. Acute confusion + cerebellar symptoms. Caution with carbamazepine. Acute confusion + cerebellar symptoms.			
Sodium valproate Depakote	3–5 h	- glucuronidation - mitochondrial oxidation - CYP2C9, CYP2A6	—	8–20 h 14 h
	Contraindicated in patients with active liver disease, personal or family history of severe hepatic dysfunction, drug related and porphyria. Effects of valproate on other drugs: Valproate decreases the metabolism of lamotrigine. Potential for lamotrigine toxicity (See below). Valproate decreases the metabolism of zidovudine. Potential for zidovudine toxicity. Valproate displaces warfarin from plasma proteins. Monitor PTT. Effects of other drugs on valproate: Carbamazepine, mefloquine, chloroquine, carbapenem antibiotics and rifampicin can decrease plasma valproate levels. Aspirin displaces valproate from plasma proteins, increasing valproate levels. Valproate + topiramate. Potential for encephalopathy, hyperammonemia.			
Lamotrigine	2.5 h	- glucuronidation	—	33 h (14–103 h)
	Caution in renal impairment. Reduce initiation, escalation and maintenance doses of lamotrigine. Valproate decreases the metabolism of lamotrigine. Potential for lamotrigine toxicity. Reduce lamotrigine initiation and escalation doses by 50%. Start lamotrigine at 25 mg alternate day dosing for the first 14 days. Carbamazepine, rifampicin, lopinavir/ritonavir increase the metabolism of lamotrigine. Increase lamotrigine initiation and escalation doses. Start lamotrigine at 50 mg d^{-1} dosing for the first 14 days. Hormonal contraceptives containing ethinyloestradiol/levonorgestrel combination increase the clearance of lamotrigine twofold. Following titration, higher maintenance doses of lamotrigine may be needed.			
Carbamazepine	12 h by 24 h (prolonged release)	- CYP3A4 - epoxide hydrolase	carbamazepine 10, 11-epoxide	16–24 h

Drug	Time to peak plasma concentration t_max	Metabolism	Active metabolite	Half-life t_½

Contraindications: AV block, history of bone marrow depression, or hepatic porphyria.

Carbamazepine + MAOI contraindicated. Need 14/7 MAOI washout.

Avoid clozapine + carbamazepine combination. ↑ risk of agranulocytosis.

Carbamazepine is a potent inducer of CYP3A4 and other phase I and phase II liver enzyme systems.

With repeated dosing, carbamazepine induces its own metabolism.

Effects of carbamazepine on other drugs:

Carbamazepine can result in the failure of oral contraceptives containing oestrogen and/or progesterone.

Carbamazepine can lower the plasma concentrations and lead to treatment failure with: buprenorphine, methadone, warfarin, bupropion, citalopram, sertraline, trazodone, imipramine, amitriptyline, nortriptyline, clomipramine, levothyroxine, lamotrigine, valproate, haloperidol, olanzapine, quetiapine, risperidone, aripiprazole, paliperidone, alprazolam, protease inhibitors, theophylline, dihydropyridines, digoxin, statins, ivabradine, corticosteroids, and immunosuppressants.

Effects of other drugs on carbamazepine:

Inducers and inhibitors of CYP3A4 can decrease and increase plasma carbamazepine concentrations respectively.

The following can increase plasma carbamazepine concentrations: fluoxetine, fluvoxamine, paroxetine, trazodone, loratadine, olanzapine, ritonavir, diltiazem. Potential for carbamazepine toxicity: cerebellar symptoms/signs, diplopia drowsiness.

The following can increase plasma carbamazepine concentrations: St John's wort, modafinil, isotretinoin, theophylline, aminophylline.

Specific interactions:

Diuretic + carbamazepine. Potential for hyponatremia.

Antipsychotic or lithium + carbamazepine. Potential for neurotoxicity.

CYP2D6 inhibitors fluoxetine, paroxetine, bupropion, duloxetine promethazine quinidine ritonavir	*Weak CYP2D6 inducers* carbamazepine rifampicin
CYP3A4 inhibitors fluoxetine, paroxetine erythromycin, clarithromycin ketoconazole, itraconazole ritonavir grapefruit juice	*CYP3A4 inducers* carbamazepine, phenytoin St John's wort modafinil
CYP1A2 inhibitors fluvoxamine ciprofloxacin verapamil erythromycin caffeine	*CYP1A2 inducers* tobacco modafinil phenytoin omeprazole rifampicin

Source: Data from electronic medicines compendium (EMC). https://www.medicines.org.uk/emc/.

Appendix 2

The metabolic syndrome

Measure	Value
Waist circumference	male ≥94 cm, 37 in.; female ≥80 cm, 31.5 in.
High density lipoprotein (HDL)	male <1.03 mmol l^{-1}; female <1.29 mmol l^{-1}
Triglycerides	≥1.7 mmol l^{-1}
Glucose dysregulation	>5.5 mmol l^{-1} (*fasting blood glucose*)
Blood pressure	≥130/85 mmHg

Waist criteria + 2 others = metabolic syndrome.

Advanced Prescribing in Psychosis, First Edition. Paul Morrison, David M. Taylor and Phillip McGuire.
© 2020 John Wiley & Sons Ltd. Published 2020 by John Wiley & Sons Ltd.

Physical health monitoring for patients prescribed antipsychotics

Measure	At baseline	Initiation phase	At 3 month stage	Every 6 months	Annually
Weight	x	Weekly for 6 weeks		x	

Nutrition risk screening at baseline.
Advice & information on cardioprotective diet at NHS Choices: http://www.nhs.uk/Livewell/healthy-eating/Pages/Healthyeating.aspx
Referral to dietitian?
Exercise. Physical activity guidelines for adults at NHS Choices: http://www.nhs.uk/Livewell/fitness/Pages/physical-activity-guidelines-for-adults.aspx

Measure	At baseline	Initiation phase	At 3 month stage	Every 6 months	Annually
Waist circumference	x		x		x
Smoking status	x				x

Nicotine replacement therapy should be considered as first-line pharmacotherapy. There are multiple preparations, and all routes of administration are effective at ameliorating symptoms of withdrawal and are associated with improved rates of smoking cessation. Dosages will vary according to the degree of nicotine dependence. Simultaneous use of long- (e.g. patch) and intermittent short-acting formulations (e.g. spray) appear to be more effective, and duration of treatment can last 8–12 weeks [385].
second-line: varenicline, bupropion.

Measure	At baseline	Initiation phase	At 3 month stage	Every 6 months	Annually
Diabetes screening ■ Fasting blood glucose ■ Hb1Ac	x	Monthly for 3 months on clozapine or olanzapine	x		x
Lipids	x		x		x
Blood pressure/pulse	x		x		x
Temperature	x		x		x
Full physical examination	x				x

(Continued)

Advanced Prescribing in Psychosis, First Edition. Paul Morrison, David M. Taylor and Phillip McGuire.
© 2020 John Wiley & Sons Ltd. Published 2020 by John Wiley & Sons Ltd.

Measure	At baseline	Initiation phase	At 3 month stage	Every 6 months	Annually
Extra-pyramidal signs, especially if: ■ high-potency D$_2$ drug.	x	Weekly for 6 weeks	x		
ECG if: ■ Inpatients ■ Personal or family history of CVS disease. ■ Risk factors for long QTc. ■ Hypertension. ■ Haloperidol, clozapine.	x				x
U&E's, FBC, LFTs	x				x
CK, prolactin	x				

Physical health monitoring for patients prescribed mood stabilisers

Drug	Plasma level	Baseline checks	Ongoing checks
Lithium carbonate	3–5 days after initiation or dose change Sample at 12 h post-dose. Target (mmol l^{-1}) ■ Maintenance 0.6–0.8 ■ In mania up to 1.2	■ Renal function ■ Ca^{2+} ■ TFTs ■ FBC ■ Weight ■ ECG if history of CVS disease or risk factors ■ Weight	Every 3 months ■ Li$^+$ plasma level Every 6 months: ■ TFTs ■ renal function ■ Ca^{2+} ■ Weight
Mild/moderate renal insufficiency: monitor Li$^+$ plasma levels closely. ■ Toxicity: plasma levels of 1.5 mmol l^{-1}. ■ NSAIDs, ACE inhibitors, diuretics, steroids, tetracyclines can ↑ Li$^+$ plasma levels. ■ Avoid dehydration. See drug interactions, Appendix			
Valproate	Titrate dose versus response and tolerability. Sample at trough. Target (mg l^{-1}) ■ Maintenance 50–100 ■ In mania up to 125	■ FBC ■ LFTs ■ Prothrombin rate	Every 3 months ■ Weight Every 6 months: ■ FBC ■ LFTs ■ Prothrombin rate
Transient increased transaminases are common at the beginning of treatment. Low prothrombin rate: cessation of valproate. Liaise with physicians. Nausea/vomiting, acute abdominal pain. Need serum amylase. See drug interactions, Appendix			
Lamotrigine	Target (mg l^{-1}) ■ not established	nil	nil

(Continued)

Advanced Prescribing in Psychosis, First Edition. Paul Morrison, David M. Taylor and Phillip McGuire.
© 2020 John Wiley & Sons Ltd. Published 2020 by John Wiley & Sons Ltd.

Drug	Plasma level	Baseline checks	Ongoing checks
See drug interactions, Appendix			
Carbamazepine	14 days after initiation or dose change Sample at trough. Target (mg l⁻¹) epilepsy 4–12 mg l⁻¹ bipolar >7 mg l⁻¹ (?)	■ FBC ■ LFTs ■ Renal function ■ Weight	Every 6 months: ■ Carbamazepine plasma level ■ FBC ■ LFTs ■ Renal function ■ Weight

Increase in GGT, Alk phos due to enzyme induction. Not an indication for cessation of carbamazepine.

Check HLA-B-*1502 allele in individuals of Han Chinese, Thai, Philippines, Malaysian origin. High risk of Stevens-Johnson syndrome in +ve carriers.

Careful monitoring of plasma Na^+ if pre-existing renal condition or medications associated with hyponatremia (e.g. diuretics).

See drug interactions, Appendix

References

1. Turner, J., Hayward, R., Angel, K. et al. (2015). The history of mental health services in modern England: practitioner memories and the direction of future research. Med. Hist. 59 (4): 599–624.
2. Wing, J.K., Cooper, J.E., and Sartorius, N. (1974). Measurement and Classification of Psychiatric Symptoms; An Instruction Manual for the PSE and Catego Program. Cambridge University Press.
3. Ayesa-Arriola, R., Moríñigo, J.D.L., David, A.S. et al. (2014). Lack of insight 3 years after first-episode psychosis: an unchangeable illness trait determined from first presentation? Schizophr. Res. 157 (1–3): 271–277.
4. David, A., Fleminger, S., Kopelman, M. et al. (2016). Wiley: Lishman's Organic Psychiatry: A Textbook of Neuropsychiatry, 4e. Available from: http://eu.wiley.com/WileyCDA/WileyTitle/productCd-0470675071.html.
5. Murray, R.M., Paparelli, A., Morrison, P.D. et al. (2013). What can we learn about schizophrenia from studying the human model, drug-induced psychosis? Am. J. Med. Genet. B Neuropsychiatr. Genet. 162B (7): 661–670.
6. Tulloch, A.D., Frayn, E., Craig, T.K.J., and Nicholson, T.R.J. (2012). Khat use among Somali mental health service users in South London. Soc. Psychiatry Psychiatr. Epidemiol. 47 (10): 1649–1656.
7. Engstrom, E.J. (2004). Clinical Psychiatry in Imperial Germany: A History of Psychiatric Practice. Ithaca, NY: Cornell University Press. 9780801441950 p. (Cornell Studies in the History of Psychiatry).
8. Fusar-Poli, P., Cappucciati, M., Bonoldi, I. et al. (2016). Prognosis of brief psychotic episodes: a meta-analysis. JAMA Psychiatry 73 (3): 211–220.
9. Pearse, L.J., Dibben, C., Ziauddeen, H. et al. (2014). A study of psychotic symptoms in borderline personality disorder. J. Nerv. Ment. Dis. 202 (5): 368–371.
10. Merrett, Z., Rossell, S.L., and Castle, D.J. (2016). Comparing the experience of voices in borderline personality disorder with the experience of voices in a psychotic disorder: a systematic review. Aust. N.Z.J. Psychiatry 50 (7): 640–648.
11. Oliva, F., Dalmotto, M., Pirfo, E. et al. (2014). A comparison of thought and perception disorders in borderline personality disorder and schizophrenia: psychotic experiences as a reaction to impaired social functioning. BMC Psychiatry 14: 239.
12. Stefanis, N.C., Hanssen, M., Smirnis, N.K. et al. (2002). Evidence that three dimensions of psychosis have a distribution in the general population. Psychol. Med. 32 (2): 347–358.
13. Schlier, B., Scheunemann, J., and Lincoln, T.M. (2016). Continuum beliefs about psychotic symptoms are a valid, unidimensional construct: construction and validation of a revised continuum beliefs questionnaire. Psychiatry Res. 241: 147–153.
14. Linscott, R.J. and van Os, J. (2013). An updated and conservative systematic review and meta-analysis of epidemiological evidence on psychotic experiences in children and adults: on the pathway from proneness to persistence to dimensional expression across mental disorders. Psychol. Med. 43 (6): 1133–1149.
15. van Os, J. and Murray, R.M. (2013). Can we identify and treat "schizophrenia light" to prevent true psychotic illness? BMJ 346: f304.
16. Pedrosa, D.J., Geyer, C., Klosterkötter, J. et al. (2012). Anti-NMDA receptor encephalitis: a neurological and psychiatric emergency. Fortschr. Neurol. Psychiatr. 80 (1): 29–35.
17. Craddock, N., Antebi, D., Attenburrow, M.-J. et al. (2008). Wake-up call for British psychiatry. Br. J. Psychiatry 193 (1): 6–9.
18. Queirazza, F., Semple, D.M., and Lawrie, S.M. (2014). Transition to schizophrenia in acute and transient psychotic disorders. Br. J. Psychiatry 204: 299–305.
19. Andreasen, N.C. and Carpenter, W.T. (1993). Diagnosis and classification of schizophrenia. Schizophr. Bull. 19 (2): 199–214.
20. Bleuler, E. (1911). Dementia praecox oder Gruppe der Schizophrenien, Handbuch der Psychiatrie. Leipzig: Deuticke [cited 2016 Jul 26]; Available from: http://ci.nii.ac.jp/naid/10014515664.

Advanced Prescribing in Psychosis, First Edition. Paul Morrison, David M. Taylor and Phillip McGuire.
© 2020 John Wiley & Sons Ltd. Published 2020 by John Wiley & Sons Ltd.

21. Kraepelin, E. (1896). Psychiatrie: ein Lehrbuch für Studirende und Aerzte (5e Auflage)/von Dr. Emil Kraepelin. Leipzig: Barth [cited 2016 Jul 26]. Available from: http://gallica.bnf.fr/ark:/12148/bpt6k76636h.

22. Kendler, K.S. (2016). The nature of psychiatric disorders. World Psychiatry 15 (1): 5–12.

23. Lasalvia, A., Penta, E., Sartorius, N., and Henderson, S. (2015). Should the label "schizophrenia" be abandoned? Schizophr. Res. 162 (1–3): 276–284.

24. van Os, J. (2016). "Schizophrenia" does not exist. BMJ 352: i375.

25. Jäger, M., Bottlender, R., Strauss, A., and Möller, H.-J. (2003). On the descriptive validity of ICD-10 schizophrenia: empirical analyses in the spectrum of non-affective functional psychoses. Psychopathology 36 (3): 152–159.

26. Carpenter, W.T., Arango, C., Buchanan, R.W., and Kirkpatrick, B. (1999). Deficit psychopathology and a paradigm shift in schizophrenia research. Biol. Psychiatry 46 (3): 352–360.

27. Malaspina, D., Walsh-Messinger, J., Gaebel, W. et al. (2014). Negative symptoms, past and present: a historical perspective and moving to DSM-5. Eur. Neuropsychopharmacol. 24 (5): 710–724.

28. Aleman, A., Lincoln, T.M., Bruggeman, R. et al. (2016). Treatment of negative symptoms: where do we stand, and where do we go? Schizophr. Res. 186: 55–62.

29. Patel, R., Jayatilleke, N., Broadbent, M. et al. (2015). Negative symptoms in schizophrenia: a study in a large clinical sample of patients using a novel automated method. BMJ Open 5 (9): e007619.

30. Forster, R. (2000). Many faces of deinstitutionalization – sociological interpretation. Psychiatr. Prax. 27 (Suppl 2): S39–S43.

31. Lamb, H.R. (1998). Deinstitutionalization at the beginning of the new millennium. Harv. Rev. Psychiatry 6 (1): 1–10.

32. de Leon, J. (2014). Paradoxes of US psychopharmacology practice in 2013: undertreatment of severe mental illness and overtreatment of minor psychiatric problems. J. Clin. Psychopharmacol. 34 (5): 545–548.

33. Grande, I., Berk, M., Birmaher, B., and Vieta, E. (2016). Bipolar disorder. Lancet 387 (10027): 1561–1572.

34. de Assis da Silva, R., Mograbi, D.C., Silveira, L.A.S. et al. (2013). Mood self-assessment in bipolar disorder: a comparison between patients in mania, depression, and euthymia. Trends Psychiatry Psychother. 35 (2): 141–145.

35. Ramachandran, A.S., Ramanathan, R., Praharaj, S.K. et al. (2016). A cross-sectional, comparative study of insight in schizophrenia and bipolar patients in remission. Indian J. Psychol. Med. 38 (3): 207–212.

36. Angst, J., Gamma, A., Bowden, C.L. et al. (2013). Evidence-based definitions of bipolar-I and bipolar-II disorders among 5,635 patients with major depressive episodes in the Bridge Study: validity and comorbidity. Eur. Arch. Psychiatry Clin. Neurosci. 263 (8): 663–673.

37. Angst, J., Ajdacic-Gross, V., and Rössler, W. (2015). Classification of mood disorders. Psychiatr. Pol. 49 (4): 663–671.

38. Murray, R.M., Morrison, P.D., Henquet, C., and Di Forti, M. (2007). Cannabis, the mind and society: the hash realities. Nat. Rev. Neurosci. 8 (11): 885–895.

39. Di Forti, M., Marconi, A., Carra, E. et al. (2015). Proportion of patients in south London with first-episode psychosis attributable to use of high potency cannabis: a case-control study. Lancet Psychiatry 2 (3): 233–238.

40. Englund, A., Morrison, P.D., Nottage, J. et al. (2013). Cannabidiol inhibits THC-elicited paranoid symptoms and hippocampal-dependent memory impairment. J. Psychopharmacol (Oxford). 27 (1): 19–27.

41. McGuire, P., Robson, P., Cubala, W.J. et al. (2018). Cannabidiol (CBD) as an adjunctive therapy in schizophrenia: a multicenter randomized controlled trial. Am. J. Psychiatry 175 (3): 225–231.

42. Morrison, P.D., Zois, V., McKeown, D.A. et al. (2009). The acute effects of synthetic intravenous Delta9-tetrahydrocannabinol on psychosis, mood and cognitive functioning. Psychol. Med. 39 (10): 1607–1616.

43. Arendt, M., Rosenberg, R., Foldager, L. et al. (2005). Cannabis-induced psychosis and subsequent schizophrenia-spectrum disorders: follow-up study of 535 incident cases. Br. J. Psychiatry 187: 510–515.

44. Niemi-Pynttäri, J.A., Sund, R., Putkonen, H. et al. (2013). Substance-induced psychoses converting into schizophrenia: a register-based study of 18,478 Finnish inpatient cases. J. Clin. Psychiatry 74 (1): e94–e99.

45. Nia, A.B., Medrano, B., Perkel, C. et al. (2016). Psychiatric comorbidity associated with synthetic cannabinoid use compared to cannabis. J. Psychopharmacol. (Oxford).

46. Tracy, D.K., Wood, D.M., and Baumeister, D. (2017). Novel psychoactive substances: types, mechanisms of action, and effects. BMJ 356: i6848.

47. Ralphs, R., Williams, L., Askew, R., and Norton, A. (2017). Adding spice to the porridge: the development of a synthetic cannabinoid market in an English prison. Int. J. Drug Policy 40: 57–69.

48. Allsop, D.J., Copeland, J., Norberg, M.M. et al. (2012 [cited 2016 Jul 26];). Quantifying the clinical significance of cannabis withdrawal. PLoS One 7 (9) Available from: http://www.ncbi.nlm.nih.gov/pmc/articles/PMC3458862/.

49. Wilkinson, S.T., Yarnell, S., Radhakrishnan, R. et al. (2016). Marijuana legalization: impact on physicians and public health. Annu. Rev. Med. 67: 453–466.

50. López-Muñoz, F., Bhatara, V.S., Alamo, C., and Cuenca, E. (2004). Historical approach to reserpine discovery and its introduction in psychiatry. Actas Esp. Psiquiatr. 32 (6): 387–395.

51. Elkes, J. (1995). Psychopharmacology: finding one's way. Neuropsychopharmacology 12 (2): 93–111.

52. Schou, M. (1997). Forty years of lithium treatment. Arch. Gen. Psychiatry 54 (1): 9–13; discussion 14–15.

53. Ackner, B., Harris, A., and Oldham, A.J. (1957). Insulin treatment of schizophrenia; a controlled study. Lancet 272 (6969): 607–611.

54. Lester, H. and Glasby, J. (2006). Mental Health: Policy and Practice, 256. Basingstoke, England; New York: Palgrave Macmillan.

55. Winkler, P., Barrett, B., McCrone, P. et al. (2016). Deinstitutionalised patients, homelessness and imprisonment: systematic review. Br. J. Psychiatry 208 (5): 421–428.

56. Harrison, P.J., Baldwin, D.S., Barnes, T.R.E. et al. (2011). No psychiatry without psychopharmacology. Br. J. Psychiatry 199 (4): 263–265.

57. Patterson, T.L. and Leeuwenkamp, O.R. (2008). Adjunctive psychosocial therapies for the treatment of schizophrenia. Schizophr. Res. 100 (1–3): 108–119.

58. Leucht, S., Cipriani, A., Spineli, L. et al. (2013). Comparative efficacy and tolerability of 15 antipsychotic drugs in schizophrenia: a multiple-treatments meta-analysis. Lancet 382 (9896): 951–962.

59. Kapur, S. and Remington, G. (2001). Dopamine D(2) receptors and their role in atypical antipsychotic action: still necessary and may even be sufficient. Biol. Psychiatry 50 (11): 873–883.

60. Nur, S. and Adams, C.E. (2016). Chlorpromazine versus reserpine for schizophrenia. Cochrane Database Syst. Rev. 4 (Art. No.: CD012122). doi: https://doi.org/10.1002/14651858.CD012122.pub2.

61. Young, S.L., Taylor, M., and Lawrie, S.M. (2015). "First do no harm." A systematic review of the prevalence and management of antipsychotic adverse effects. J. Psychopharmacol (Oxford). 29 (4): 353–362.

62. Lambert, M., Conus, P., Eide, P. et al. (2004). Impact of present and past antipsychotic side effects on attitude toward typical antipsychotic treatment and adherence. Eur. Psychiatry 19 (7): 415–422.

63. Fleischhacker, W.W., Meise, U., Günther, V., and Kurz, M. (1994). Compliance with antipsychotic drug treatment: influence of side effects. Acta Psychiatr. Scand. 382: 11–15.

64. Carpenter, W.T. (1996). Maintenance therapy of persons with schizophrenia. J. Clin. Psychiatry 57 (Suppl 9): 10–18.

65. Caseiro, O., Pérez-Iglesias, R., Mata, I. et al. (2012). Predicting relapse after a first episode of non-affective psychosis: a three-year follow-up study. J. Psychiatr. Res. 46 (8): 1099–1105.

66. Cesuroglu, T., Syurina, E., Feron, F., and Krumeich, A. (2016). Other side of the coin for personalised medicine and healthcare: content analysis of "personalised" practices in the literature. BMJ Open 6 (7): e010243.

67. Montgomery, S.A., Locklear, J.C., Svedsäter, H., and Eriksson, H. (2014). Efficacy of once-daily extended release quetiapine fumarate in patients with different levels of severity of generalized anxiety disorder. Int. Clin. Psychopharmacol. 29 (5): 252–262.

68. Veale, D., Miles, S., Smallcombe, N. et al. (2014). Atypical antipsychotic augmentation in SSRI treatment refractory obsessive-compulsive disorder: a systematic review and meta-analysis. BMC Psychiatry 14: 317.

69. Chen, J., Gao, K., and Kemp, D.E. (2011). Second-generation antipsychotics in major depressive disorder: update and clinical perspective. Curr. Opin. Psychiatry 24 (1): 10–17.

70. Urs, N.M., Nicholls, P.J., and Caron, M.G. (2014). Integrated approaches to understanding antipsychotic drug action at GPCRs. Curr. Opin. Cell Biol. 27: 56–62.

71. Kumari, P., Ghosh, E., and Shukla, A.K. (2015). Emerging approaches to GPCR ligand screening for drug discovery. Trends Mol. Med. 21 (11): 687–701.

72. Sato, H., Ito, C., Hiraoka, K. et al. (2015). Histamine H1 receptor occupancy by the new-generation antipsychotics olanzapine and quetiapine: a positron emission tomography study in healthy volunteers. Psychopharmacology (Berl) 232 (19): 3497–3505.

73. Li, M.-L., Hu, X.-Q., Li, F., and Gao, W.-J. (2015). Perspectives on the mGluR2/3 agonists as a therapeutic target for schizophrenia: still promising or a dead end? Prog. Neuro-Psychopharmacol. Biol. Psychiatry 60: 66–76.

74. Singer, P., Dubroqua, S., and Yee, B.K. (2015). Inhibition of glycine transporter 1: the yellow brick road to new schizophrenia therapy? Curr. Pharm. Des. 21 (26): 3771–3787.

75. Siskind, D., McCartney, L., Goldschlager, R., and Kisely, S. (2016). Clozapine v. first- and second-generation antipsychotics in treatment-refractory schizophrenia: systematic review and meta-analysis. Br. J. Psychiatry.

76. Lieberman, J.A. (2007). Effectiveness of antipsychotic drugs in patients with chronic schizophrenia: efficacy, safety and cost outcomes of CATIE and other trials. J. Clin. Psychiatry 68 (2): e04.

77. Jones, P.B., Barnes, T.R.E., Davies, L. et al. (2006). Randomized controlled trial of the effect on quality of life of second- vs first-generation antipsychotic drugs in schizophrenia: cost utility of the latest antipsychotic drugs in schizophrenia study (CUtLASS 1). Arch. Gen. Psychiatry 63 (10): 1079–1087.

78. Kahn, R.S., Fleischhacker, W.W., Boter, H. et al. (2008). Effectiveness of antipsychotic drugs in first-episode schizophrenia and schizophreniform disorder: an open randomised clinical trial. Lancet 371 (9618): 1085–1097.

79. Agid, O., Arenovich, T., Sajeev, G. et al. (2011). An algorithm-based approach to first-episode schizophrenia: response rates over 3 prospective antipsychotic trials with a retrospective data analysis. J. Clin. Psychiatry 72 (11): 1439–1444.

80. Attard, A. and Taylor, D.M. (2012). Comparative effectiveness of atypical antipsychotics in schizophrenia: what have real-world trials taught us? CNS Drugs 26 (6): 491–508.

81. Batail, J.-M., Langrée, B., Robert, G. et al. (2014). Use of very-high-dose olanzapine in treatment-resistant schizophrenia. Schizophr. Res. 159 (2–3): 411–414.

82. Carpenter, W.T. and Buchanan, R.W. (2008). Lessons to take home from CATIE. Psychiatr. Serv. 59 (5): 523–525.

83. Meltzer, H.Y. and Massey, B.W. (2011). The role of serotonin receptors in the action of atypical antipsychotic drugs. Curr. Opin. Pharmacol. 11 (1): 59–67.

84. Voicu, V., Medvedovici, A., Ranetti, A.E., and Rădulescu, F.Ş. (2013). Drug-induced hypo- and hyperprolactinemia: mechanisms, clinical and therapeutic consequences. Expert Opin. Drug Metab. Toxicol. 9 (8): 955–968.

85. Citrome, L., Kalsekar, I., Baker, R.A., and Hebden, T. (2014). A review of real-world data on the effects of aripiprazole on weight and metabolic outcomes in adults. Curr. Med. Res. Opin. 30 (8): 1629–1641.

86. Meyer, J.M., Mao, Y., Pikalov, A. et al. (2015). Weight change during long-term treatment with lurasidone: pooled analysis of studies in patients with schizophrenia. Int. Clin. Psychopharmacol. 30 (6): 342–350.

87. Haddad, P.M. and Sharma, S.G. (2007). Adverse effects of atypical antipsychotics: differential risk and clinical implications. CNS Drugs 21 (11): 911–936.

88. Kelly, D.L., Conley, R.R., and Carpenter, W.T. (2005). First-episode schizophrenia: a focus on pharmacological treatment and safety considerations. Drugs 65 (8): 1113–1138.

89. Shayegan, D.K. and Stahl, S.M. (2004). Atypical antipsychotics: matching receptor profile to individual patient's clinical profile. CNS Spectr. 9 (10 Suppl 11): 6–14.

90. Naber, D. and Lambert, M. (2009). The CATIE and CUtLASS studies in schizophrenia: results and implications for clinicians. CNS Drugs 23 (8): 649–659.

91. Friis, S., Melle, I., Johannessen, J.O. et al. (2016). Early predictors of ten-year course in first-episode psychosis. Psychiatr. Serv. 67 (4): 438–443.

92. Souaiby, L., Gaillard, R., and Krebs, M.-O. (2016). Duration of untreated psychosis: a state-of-the-art review and critical analysis. Encephale 42 (4): 361–366.

93. Díaz-Caneja, C.M., Pina-Camacho, L., Rodríguez-Quiroga, A. et al. (2015). Predictors of outcome in early-onset psychosis: a systematic review. NPJ Schizophr. 1: 14005.

94. Alvarez, E., Bobes, J., Gómez, J.-C. et al. (2003). Safety of olanzapine versus conventional antipsychotics in the treatment of patients with acute schizophrenia. A naturalistic study. Eur. Neuropsychopharmacol. 13 (1): 39–48.

95. Cañas, F., Ciudad, A., Gutiérrez, M. et al. (2005). Safety, effectiveness, and patterns of use of olanzapine in acute schizophrenia: a multivariate analysis of a large naturalistic study in the hospital setting. Med. Clin (Barc). 124 (13): 481–486.

96. Tarricone, I., Ferrari Gozzi, B., Serretti, A. et al. (2010). Weight gain in antipsychotic-naive patients: a review and meta-analysis. Psychol. Med. 40 (2): 187–200.

97. Tek, C., Kucukgoncu, S., Guloksuz, S. et al. (2016). Antipsychotic-induced weight gain in first-episode psychosis patients: a meta-analysis of differential effects of antipsychotic medications. Early Interv. Psychiatry 10 (3): 193–202.

98. Rado, J. and von Ammon Cavanaugh, S. (2016). A naturalistic randomized placebo-controlled trial of extended-release metformin to prevent weight gain associated with olanzapine in a US community-dwelling population. J. Clin. Psychopharmacol. 36 (2): 163–168.

99. Larsen, J.R., Vedtofte, L., Jakobsen, M.S.L. et al. (2017). Effect of liraglutide treatment on prediabetes and overweight or obesity in clozapine- or olanzapine-treated patients with schizophrenia spectrum disorder: a randomized clinical trial. JAMA Psychiatry 74 (7): 719–728.

100. Wang, L.-J., Ree, S.-C., Huang, Y.-S. et al. (2013). Adjunctive effects of aripiprazole on metabolic profiles: comparison of patients treated with olanzapine to patients treated with other atypical antipsychotic drugs. Prog. Neuro-Psychopharmacol. Biol. Psychiatry 40: 260–266.

101. Howard, R., Cort, E., Bradley, R. et al. (2018). Antipsychotic treatment of very late-onset schizophrenia-like psychosis (ATLAS): a randomised, controlled, double-blind trial. Lancet Psychiatry 5 (7): 553–563.

102. Samara, M.T., Leucht, C., Leeflang, M.M. et al. (2015). Early improvement as a predictor of later response to antipsychotics in schizophrenia: a diagnostic test review. Am. J. Psychiatry 172 (7): 617–629.

103. Dold, M. and Leucht, S. (2014). Pharmacotherapy of treatment-resistant schizophrenia: a clinical perspective. Evid. Based Ment. Health 17 (2): 33–37.

104. Taylor, D., Paton, C., and Kapur, S. (2015). The Maudsley Prescribing Guidelines in Psychiatry. 12 Rev. ed., 760. Chichester, West Sussex; Hoboken, NJ: Wiley-Blackwell.

105. Bitter, I., Fehér, L., Tényi, T., and Czobor, P. (2015). Treatment adherence and insight in schizophrenia. Psychiatr. Hung. 30 (1): 18–26.

106. Novick, D., Montgomery, W., Treuer, T. et al. (2015). Relationship of insight with medication adherence and the impact on outcomes in patients with schizophrenia and bipolar disorder: results from a 1-year European outpatient observational study. BMC Psychiatry 15: 189.

107. Czobor, P., Van Dorn, R.A., Citrome, L. et al. (2015). Treatment adherence in schizophrenia: a patient-level meta-analysis of combined CATIE and EUFEST studies. Eur. Neuropsychopharmacol. 25 (8): 1158–1166.

108. Drake, R.J., Nordentoft, M., Haddock, G. et al. (2015). Modeling determinants of medication attitudes and poor adherence in early nonaffective psychosis: implications for intervention. Schizophr. Bull. 41 (3): 584–596.

109. Drake, R.J., Dunn, G., Tarrier, N. et al. (2007). Insight as a predictor of the outcome of first-episode nonaffective psychosis in a prospective cohort study in England. J. Clin. Psychiatry 68 (1): 81–86.

110. Perkins, D.O., Johnson, J.L., Hamer, R.M. et al. (2006). Predictors of antipsychotic medication adherence in patients recovering from a first psychotic episode. Schizophr. Res. 83 (1): 53–63.

111. Ascher-Svanum, H., Faries, D.E., Zhu, B. et al. (2006). Medication adherence and long-term functional outcomes in the treatment of schizophrenia in usual care. J. Clin. Psychiatry 67 (3): 453–460.

112. Dunayevich, E., Ascher-Svanum, H., Zhao, F. et al. (2007). Longer time to antipsychotic treatment discontinuation for any cause is associated with better functional outcomes for patients with schizophrenia, schizophreniform disorder, or schizoaffective disorder. J. Clin. Psychiatry 68 (8): 1163–1171.

113. Robinson, D., Woerner, M.G., Alvir, J.M. et al. (1999). Predictors of relapse following response from a first episode of schizophrenia or schizoaffective disorder. Arch. Gen. Psychiatry 56 (3): 241–247.

114. Alvarez-Jimenez, M., Priede, A., Hetrick, S.E. et al. (2012). Risk factors for relapse following treatment for first episode psychosis: a systematic review and meta-analysis of longitudinal studies. Schizophr. Res. 139 (1–3): 116–128.

115. Zipursky, R.B., Menezes, N.M., and Streiner, D.L. (2014). Risk of symptom recurrence with medication discontinuation in first-episode psychosis: a systematic review. Schizophr. Res. 152 (2–3): 408–414.

116. Winton-Brown, T.T., Elanjithara, T., Power, P. et al. (2017). Five-fold increased risk of relapse following breaks in antipsychotic treatment of first episode psychosis. Schizophr. Res. 179: 50–56.

117. Lieberman, J.A., Alvir, J.M., Koreen, A. et al. (1996). Psychobiologic correlates of treatment response in schizophrenia. Neuropsychopharmacology 14 (3 Suppl): 13S–21S.

118. Emsley, R., Chiliza, B., Asmal, L., and Harvey, B.H. (2013). The nature of relapse in schizophrenia. BMC Psychiatry 13: 50.

119. Lally, J. and MacCabe, J.H. (2015). Antipsychotic medication in schizophrenia: a review. Br. Med. Bull. 114 (1): 169–179.

120. Cowen, P.J. (2011). Has psychopharmacology got a future? Br. J. Psychiatry 198 (5): 333–335.

121. Gray, R., Bressington, D., Ivanecka, A. et al. (2016). Is adherence therapy an effective adjunct treatment for patients with schizophrenia spectrum disorders? A systematic review and meta-analysis. BMC Psychiatry 16: 90.

122. Kopelowicz, A., Zarate, R., Wallace, C.J. et al. (2012). The ability of multifamily groups to improve treatment adherence in Mexican Americans with schizophrenia. Arch. Gen. Psychiatry 69 (3): 265–273.

123. Chien, W.T., Mui, J.H.C., Cheung, E.F.C., and Gray, R. (2015). Effects of motivational interviewing-based adherence therapy for schizophrenia spectrum disorders: a randomized controlled trial. Trials 16: 270.

124. von Bormann, S., Robson, D., and Gray, R. (2015). Adherence therapy following acute exacerbation of schizophrenia: a randomised controlled trial in Thailand. Int. J. Soc. Psychiatry 61 (1): 3–9.

125. MacDonald, L., Chapman, S., Syrett, M. et al. (2016). Improving medication adherence in bipolar disorder: a systematic review and meta-analysis of 30 years of intervention trials. J. Affective Disord. 194: 202–221.

126. Moran, K. and Priebe, S. (2016). Better quality of life in patients offered financial incentives for taking anti-psychotic medication: linked to improved adherence or more money? Qual. Life Res. 25 (8): 1897–1902.

127. Predmore, Z.S., Mattke, S., and Horvitz-Lennon, M. (2015). Improving antipsychotic adherence among patients with schizophrenia: savings for states. Psychiatr. Serv. 66 (4): 343–345.

128. Dilokthornsakul, P., Thoopputra, T., Patanaprateep, O. et al. (2016). Effects of medication adherence on hospitalizations and healthcare costs in patients with schizophrenia in Thailand. SAGE Open Med. 4: 2050312116637026.

129. Harrow, M. and Jobe, T.H. (2013). Does long-term treatment of schizophrenia with antipsychotic medications facilitate recovery? Schizophr. Bull. 39 (5): 962–965.

130. Tiihonen, J., Tanskanen, A., and Taipale, H. (2018). 20-year nationwide follow-up study on discontinuation of antipsychotic treatment in first-episode schizophrenia. Am. J. Psychiatry 175 (8): 765–773. appiajp201817091001.

131. Hui, C.L.M., Honer, W.G., Lee, E.H.M. et al. (2018). Long-term effects of discontinuation from antipsychotic maintenance following first-episode schizophrenia and related disorders: a 10 year follow-up of a randomised, double-blind trial. Lancet Psychiatry 5 (5): 432–442.

132. Wunderink, L., Nienhuis, F.J., Sytema, S. et al. (2007). Guided discontinuation versus maintenance treatment in remitted first-episode psychosis: relapse rates and functional outcome. J. Clin. Psychiatry 68 (5): 654–661.

133. Alvarez-Jimenez, M., O'Donoghue, B., Thompson, A. et al. (2016). Beyond clinical remission in first episode psychosis: thoughts on antipsychotic maintenance vs. guided discontinuation in the functional recovery era. CNS Drugs 30 (5): 357–368.

134. Crocq, M.-A. (2015). A history of antipsychotic long-acting injections in the treatment of schizophrenia. Encephale 41 (1): 84–92.

135. Bitter, I., Katona, L., Zámbori, J. et al. (2013). Comparative effectiveness of depot and oral second generation antipsychotic drugs in schizophrenia: a nationwide study in Hungary. Eur. Neuropsychopharmacol. 23 (11): 1383–1390.

136. Novick, D., Haro, J.M., Bertsch, J. et al. (2012). Comparison of treatment discontinuation and hospitalization among nonadherent patients initiating depot or oral typical antipsychotic medications. Int. Clin. Psychopharmacol. 27 (5): 275–282.

137. Breit, S. and Hasler, G. (2016). Advantages and controversies of depot antipsychotics in the treatment of patients with schizophrenia. Nervenarzt 87 (7): 719–723.

138. Tiihonen, J., Haukka, J., Taylor, M. et al. (2011). A nationwide cohort study of oral and depot antipsychotics after first hospitalization for schizophrenia. Am. J. Psychiatry 168 (6): 603–609.

139. Brissos, S., Veguilla, M.R., Taylor, D., and Balanzá-Martinez, V. (2014). The role of long-acting injectable antipsychotics in schizophrenia: a critical appraisal. Ther. Adv. Psychopharmacol. 4 (5): 198–219.

140. Tiihonen, J., Mittendorfer-Rutz, E., Majak, M. et al. (2017). Real-world effectiveness of antipsychotic treatments in a nationwide cohort of 29 823 patients with schizophrenia. JAMA Psychiatry 74 (7): 686–693.

141. Subotnik, K.L., Casaus, L.R., Ventura, J. et al. (2015). Long-acting injectable risperidone for relapse prevention and control of breakthrough symptoms after a recent first episode of schizophrenia. A randomized clinical trial. JAMA Psychiatry 72 (8): 822–829.

142. Patel, M.X., Nikolaou, V., and David, A.S. (2003). Psychiatrists' attitudes to maintenance medication for patients with schizophrenia. Psychol. Med. 33 (1): 83–89.

143. Meyer, J.M. (2013). Understanding depot antipsychotics: an illustrated guide to kinetics. CNS Spectr. 18 (Suppl 1): 58–67; quiz 68.

144. Kapur, S. (1998). A new framework for investigating antipsychotic action in humans: lessons from PET imaging. Mol. Psychiatry 3 (2): 135–140.

145. Gopal, S., Liu, Y., Alphs, L. et al. (2013). Incidence and time course of extrapyramidal symptoms with oral and long-acting injectable paliperidone: a posthoc pooled analysis of seven randomized controlled studies. Neuropsychiatr. Dis. Treat. 9: 1381–1392.

146. Wang, S.-M., Han, C., Lee, S.-J. et al. (2014). Schizophrenia relapse and the clinical usefulness of once-monthly aripiprazole depot injection. Neuropsychiatr. Dis. Treat. 10: 1605–1611.

147. Kane, J., Honigfeld, G., Singer, J., and Meltzer, H. (1988). Clozapine for the treatment-resistant schizophrenic. A double-blind comparison with chlorpromazine. Arch. Gen. Psychiatry 45 (9): 789–796.

148. Meltzer, H.Y. (2013). Update on typical and atypical antipsychotic drugs. Annu. Rev. Med. 64: 393–406.

149. McCutcheon, R., Beck, K., Bloomfield, M.A.P. et al. (2015). Treatment resistant or resistant to treatment? Antipsychotic plasma levels in patients with poorly controlled psychotic symptoms. J. Psychopharmacol (Oxford). 29 (8): 892–897.

150. Meltzer, H.Y., Alphs, L., Green, A.I. et al. (2003). Clozapine treatment for suicidality in schizophrenia: international suicide prevention trial (InterSePT). Arch. Gen. Psychiatry 60 (1): 82–91.

151. Meltzer, H.Y. and Okayli, G. (1995). Reduction of suicidality during clozapine treatment of neuroleptic-resistant schizophrenia: impact on risk-benefit assessment. Am. J. Psychiatry 152 (2): 183–190.

152. Victoroff, J., Coburn, K., Reeve, A. et al. (2014). Pharmacological management of persistent hostility and aggression in persons with schizophrenia spectrum disorders: a systematic review. J. Neuropsychiatry Clin. Neurosci. 26 (4): 283–312.

153. Connolly, B.S. and Lang, A.E. (2014). Pharmacological treatment of Parkinson disease: a review. JAMA 311 (16): 1670–1683.

154. Grover, S., Hazari, N., Kate, N. et al. (2014). Management of tardive syndromes with clozapine: a case series. Asian J. Psychiatry 8: 111–114.

155. Agid, O., Remington, G., Kapur, S. et al. (2007). Early use of clozapine for poorly responding first-episode psychosis. J. Clin. Psychopharmacol. 27 (4): 369–373.

156. O'Brien, A. (2004). Starting clozapine in the community: a UK perspective. CNS Drugs 18 (13): 845–852.

157. Beck, K., McCutcheon, R., Bloomfield, M.A.P. et al. (2014). The practical management of refractory schizophrenia – the Maudsley treatment review and assessment team service approach. Acta Psychiatr. Scand. 130 (6): 427–438.

158. Breslin, N.A. (1992). Treatment of schizophrenia: current practice and future promise. Hosp. Community Psychiatry 43 (9): 877–885.

159. Carpenter, W.T., Conley, R.R., Buchanan, R.W. et al. (1995). Patient response and resource management: another view of clozapine treatment of schizophrenia. Am. J. Psychiatry 152 (6): 827–832.

160. Tiihonen, J., Wahlbeck, K., and Kiviniemi, V. (2009). The efficacy of lamotrigine in clozapine-resistant schizophrenia: a systematic review and meta-analysis. Schizophr. Res. 109 (1–3): 10–14.

161. Zheng, W., Xiang, Y.-T., Xiang, Y.-Q. et al. (2016). Efficacy and safety of adjunctive topiramate for schizophrenia: a meta-analysis of randomized controlled trials. Acta Psychiatr. Scand. 134 (5): 385–398.

162. Taylor, D.M., Smith, L., Gee, S.H., and Nielsen, J. (2012). Augmentation of clozapine with a second antipsychotic – a meta-analysis. Acta Psychiatr. Scand. 125 (1): 15–24.

163. Porcelli, S., Balzarro, B., and Serretti, A. (2012). Clozapine resistance: augmentation strategies. Eur. Neuropsychopharmacol. 22 (3): 165–182.

164. Srisurapanont, M., Suttajit, S., Maneeton, N., and Maneeton, B. (2015). Efficacy and safety of aripiprazole augmentation of clozapine in schizophrenia: a systematic review and meta-analysis of randomized-controlled trials. J. Psychiatr. Res. 62: 38–47.

165. Wang, J., Omori, I.M., Fenton, M., and Soares, B. (2010). Sulpiride augmentation for schizophrenia. Cochrane Database Syst. Rev. 1 (Art. No.: CD008125). doi: https://doi.org/10.1002/14651858.CD008125.pub2.

166. Veerman, S.R.T., Schulte, P.F.J., Smith, J.D., and de Haan, L. (2016). Memantine augmentation in clozapine-refractory schizophrenia: a randomized, double-blind, placebo-controlled crossover study. Psychol. Med. 46 (9): 1909–1921.

167. de Lucena, D., Fernandes, B.S., Berk, M. et al. (2009). Improvement of negative and positive symptoms in treatment-refractory schizophrenia: a double-blind, randomized, placebo-controlled trial with memantine as add-on therapy to clozapine. J. Clin. Psychiatry 70 (10): 1416–1423.

168. Peet, M. and Horrobin, D.F. (2002). E-E Multicentre Study Group. A dose-ranging exploratory study of the effects of ethyl-eicosapentaenoate in patients with persistent schizophrenic symptoms. J. Psychiatr. Res. 36 (1): 7–18.

169. Lally, J., Tully, J., Robertson, D. et al. (2016). Augmentation of clozapine with electroconvulsive therapy in treatment resistant schizophrenia: a systematic review and meta-analysis. Schizophr. Res. 171 (1–3): 215–224.

170. Petrides, G., Malur, C., Braga, R.J. et al. (2015). Electroconvulsive therapy augmentation in clozapine-resistant schizophrenia: a prospective, randomized study. Am. J. Psychiatry 172 (1): 52–58.

171. Hynes, C., Keating, D., McWilliams, S. et al. (2015). Glasgow antipsychotic side-effects scale for clozapine – development and validation of a clozapine-specific side-effects scale. Schizophr. Res. 168 (1–2): 505–513.

172. Legge, S.E., Hamshere, M., Hayes, R.D. et al. (2016). Reasons for discontinuing clozapine: a cohort study of patients commencing treatment. Schizophr. Res. 174 (1–3): 113–119.

173. Hayes, R.D., Downs, J., Chang, C.-K. et al. (2015). The effect of clozapine on premature mortality: an assessment of clinical monitoring and other potential confounders. Schizophr. Bull. 41 (3): 644–655.

174. Lowe, C.M., Grube, R.R.A., and Scates, A.C. (2007). Characterization and clinical management of clozapine-induced fever. Ann. Pharmacother. 41 (10): 1700–1704.

175. Pui-yin Chung, J., Shiu-yin Chong, C., Chung, K. et al. (2008). The incidence and characteristics of clozapine-induced fever in a local psychiatric unit in Hong Kong. Can. J. Psychiatry 53 (12): 857–862.

176. Leung, J.Y.T., Barr, A.M., Procyshyn, R.M. et al. (2012). Cardiovascular side-effects of antipsychotic drugs: the role of the autonomic nervous system. Pharmacol. Ther. 135 (2): 113–122.

177. Lieberman, J.A. (1998). Maximizing clozapine therapy: managing side effects. J. Clin. Psychiatry 59 (Suppl 3): 38–43.

178. Merrill, D.B., Dec, G.W., and Goff, D.C. (2005). Adverse cardiac effects associated with clozapine. J. Clin. Psychopharmacol. 25 (1): 32–41.

179. Stryjer, R., Timinsky, I., Reznik, I. et al. (2009). Beta-adrenergic antagonists for the treatment of clozapine-induced sinus tachycardia: a retrospective study. Clin. Neuropharmacol. 32 (5): 290–292.

180. Lally, J., Brook, J., Dixon, T. et al. (2014). Ivabradine, a novel treatment for clozapine-induced sinus tachycardia: a case series. Ther. Adv. Psychopharmacol. 4 (3): 117–122.

181. Ronaldson, K.J., Fitzgerald, P.B., and McNeil, J.J. (2015). Clozapine-induced myocarditis, a widely overlooked adverse reaction. Acta Psychiatr. Scand. 132 (4): 231–240.

182. Ronaldson, K.J., Fitzgerald, P.B., Taylor, A.J. et al. (2011). A new monitoring protocol for clozapine-induced myocarditis based on an analysis of 75 cases and 94 controls. Aust. N.Z. J. Psychiatry 45 (6): 458–465.

183. Murch, S., Tran, N., Liew, D. et al. (2013). Echocardiographic monitoring for clozapine cardiac toxicity: lessons from real-world experience. Australas Psychiatry 21 (3): 258–261.

184. Alawami, M., Wasywich, C., Cicovic, A., and Kenedi, C. (2014). A systematic review of clozapine induced cardiomyopathy. Int. J. Cardiol. 176 (2): 315–320.

185. Watt, M.L., Rorick-Kehn, L., Shaw, D.B. et al. (2013). The muscarinic acetylcholine receptor agonist BuTAC mediates antipsychotic-like effects via the M4 subtype. Neuropsychopharmacology 38 (13): 2717–2726.

186. Olianas, M.C., Maullu, C., and Onali, P. (1997). Effects of clozapine on rat striatal muscarinic receptors coupled to inhibition of adenylyl cyclase activity and on the human cloned m4 receptor. Br. J. Pharmacol. 122 (3): 401–408.

187. Olianas, M.C., Maullu, C., and Onali, P. (1999). Mixed agonist-antagonist properties of clozapine at different human cloned muscarinic receptor subtypes expressed in Chinese hamster ovary cells. Neuropsychopharmacology 20 (3): 263–270.

188. Abrams, P., Andersson, K.-E., Buccafusco, J.J. et al. (2006). Muscarinic receptors: their distribution and function in body systems, and the implications for treating overactive bladder. Br. J. Pharmacol. 148 (5): 565–578.

189. Davydov, L. and Botts, S.R. (2000). Clozapine-induced hypersalivation. Ann. Pharmacother. 34: 662–665.

190. Kreinin, A., Miodownik, C., Mirkin, V. et al. (2016). Double-blind, randomized, placebo-controlled trial of metoclopramide for hypersalivation associated with clozapine. J. Clin. Psychopharmacol. 36 (3): 200–205.

191. Barnes, T.R.E., Drake, M.J., and Paton, C. (2012). Nocturnal enuresis with antipsychotic medication. Br. J. Psychiatry 200 (1): 7–9.

192. Every-Palmer, S., Inns, S.J., Grant, E., and Ellis, P.M. (2019). Effects of clozapine on the gut: cross-sectional study of delayed gastric emptying and small and large intestinal dysmotility. CNS Drugs 33 (1): 81–91.

193. Shirazi, A., Stubbs, B., Gomez, L. et al. (2016). Prevalence and predictors of clozapine-associated constipation: a systematic review and meta-analysis. Int. J. Mol. Sci. 17 (6).

194. Atkin, K., Kendall, F., Gould, D. et al. (1996). Neutropenia and agranulocytosis in patients receiving clozapine in the UK and Ireland. Br. J. Psychiatry 169 (4): 483–488.

195. Manu, P., Sarvaiya, N., Rogozea, L.M. et al. (2016). Benign ethnic neutropenia and clozapine use: a systematic review of the evidence and treatment recommendations. J. Clin. Psychiatry 77 (7): e909–e916.

196. Meyer, N., Gee, S., Whiskey, E. et al. (2015). Optimizing outcomes in clozapine rechallenge following neutropenia: a cohort analysis. J. Clin. Psychiatry 76 (11): e1410–e1416.

197. Whiskey, E., Olofinjana, O., and Taylor, D. (2011). The importance of the recognition of benign ethnic neutropenia in black patients during treatment with clozapine: case reports and database study. J. Psychopharmacol (Oxford). 25 (6): 842–845.

198. Varma, S., Bishara, D., Besag, F.M.C., and Taylor, D. (2011). Clozapine-related EEG changes and seizures: dose and plasma-level relationships. Ther. Adv. Psychopharmacol. 1 (2): 47–66.

199. Caetano, D. (2014). Use of anticonvulsants as prophylaxis for seizures in patients on clozapine. Australas Psychiatry 22 (1): 78–83.

200. Berk, M., Dodd, S., Callaly, P. et al. (2007). History of illness prior to a diagnosis of bipolar disorder or schizoaffective disorder. J. Affective Disord. 103 (1–3): 181–186.

201. Angst, J., Azorin, J.-M., Bowden, C.L. et al. (2011). Prevalence and characteristics of undiagnosed bipolar disorders in patients with a major depressive episode: the BRIDGE study. Arch. Gen. Psychiatry 68 (8): 791–798.

202. Baastrup, P.C. and Schou, M. (1967). Lithium as a prophylactic agents. Its effect against recurrent depressions and manic-depressive psychosis. Arch. Gen. Psychiatry 16 (2): 162–172.

203. Hunt, G.E., Malhi, G.S., Cleary, M. et al. (2016). Comorbidity of bipolar and substance use disorders in national surveys of general populations, 1990-2015: systematic review and meta-analysis. J. Affective Disord. 206: 321–330.

204. Cassidy, F., Ahearn, E.P., and Carroll, B.J. (2001). Substance abuse in bipolar disorder. Bipolar Disord. 3 (4): 181–188.

205. Salloum, I.M. and Thase, M.E. (2000). Impact of substance abuse on the course and treatment of bipolar disorder. Bipolar Disord. 2 (3 Pt 2): 269–280.

206. Dalton, E.J., Cate-Carter, T.D., Mundo, E. et al. (2003). Suicide risk in bipolar patients: the role of co-morbid substance use disorders. Bipolar Disord. 5 (1): 58–61.

207. Krishnan, K.R.R. (2005). Psychiatric and medical comorbidities of bipolar disorder. Psychosom. Med. 67 (1): 1–8.

208. Bayes, A., Parker, G., and Fletcher, K. (2014). Clinical differentiation of bipolar II disorder from borderline personality disorder. Curr. Opin. Psychiatry 27 (1): 14–20.

209. Paris, J. and Black, D.W. (2015). Borderline personality disorder and bipolar disorder: what is the difference and why does it matter? J. Nerv. Ment. Dis. 203 (1): 3–7.

210. Satzer, D. and Bond, D.J. (2016). Mania secondary to focal brain lesions: implications for understanding the functional neuroanatomy of bipolar disorder. Bipolar Disord. 18 (3): 205–220.

211. Pacchiarotti, I., Bond, D.J., Baldessarini, R.J. et al. (2013). The International Society for Bipolar Disorders (ISBD) task force report on antidepressant use in bipolar disorders. Am. J. Psychiatry 170 (11): 1249–1262.

212. Goodwin, G.M., Haddad, P.M., Ferrier, I.N. et al. (2016). Evidence-based guidelines for treating bipolar disorder: revised third edition recommendations from the British Association for Psychopharmacology. J. Psychopharmacol (Oxford). 30 (6): 495–553.

213. Suppes, T., Baldessarini, R.J., Faedda, G.L., and Tohen, M. (1991). Risk of recurrence following discontinuation of lithium treatment in bipolar disorder. Arch. Gen. Psychiatry 48 (12): 1082–1088.

214. Cipriani, A., Barbui, C., Salanti, G. et al. (2011). Comparative efficacy and acceptability of antimanic drugs in acute mania: a multiple-treatments meta-analysis. Lancet 378 (9799): 1306–1315.

215. Sachs, G., Chengappa, K.N.R., Suppes, T. et al. (2004). Quetiapine with lithium or divalproex for the treatment of bipolar mania: a randomized, double-blind, placebo-controlled study. Bipolar Disord. 6 (3): 213–223.

216. Ketter, T.A. (2008). Monotherapy versus combined treatment with second-generation antipsychotics in bipolar disorder. J. Clin. Psychiatry 69 (Suppl 5): 9–15.

217. Reischies, F.M., Hartikainen, J., and Berghöfer, A.M. (2002). Initial triple therapy of acute mania, adding lithium and valproate to neuroleptics. Pharmacopsychiatry 35 (6): 244–246.

218. Ifteni, P., Correll, C.U., Nielsen, J. et al. (2014). Rapid clozapine titration in treatment-refractory bipolar disorder. J. Affective Disord. 166: 168–172.

219. Calabrese, J.R., Kimmel, S.E., Woyshville, M.J. et al. (1996). Clozapine for treatment-refractory mania. Am. J. Psychiatry 153 (6): 759–764.

220. Li, X.-B., Tang, Y.-L., Wang, C.-Y., and de Leon, J. (2015). Clozapine for treatment-resistant bipolar disorder: a systematic review. Bipolar Disord. 17 (3): 235–247.

221. Riis, M.G. and Videbech, P.B. (2015). Marked effect of ECT in the treatment of mania. Ugeskr. Laeger 177 (20): 2–6.

222. Jauhar, S., McKenna, P.J., and Laws, K.R. (2016). NICE guidance on psychological treatments for bipolar disorder: searching for the evidence. Lancet Psychiatry 3 (4): 386–388. [cited 2016 Mar 6]; Available from: http://linkinghub.elsevier.com/retrieve/pii/S2215036615005453.

223. Young, A.H., Calabrese, J.R., Gustafsson, U. et al. (2013). Quetiapine monotherapy in bipolar II depression: combined data from four large, randomized studies. Int. J. Bipolar Disord. 1: 10.

224. Loebel, A., Cucchiaro, J., Silva, R. et al. (2014). Lurasidone monotherapy in the treatment of bipolar I depression: a randomized, double-blind, placebo-controlled study. Am. J. Psychiatry 171 (2): 160–168.

225. Taylor, D.M., Cornelius, V., Smith, L., and Young, A.H. (2014). Comparative efficacy and acceptability of drug treatments for bipolar depression: a multiple-treatments meta-analysis. Acta Psychiatr. Scand. 130 (6): 452–469.

226. Geddes, J.R., Gardiner, A., Rendell, J. et al. (2016). Comparative evaluation of quetiapine plus lamotrigine combination versus quetiapine monotherapy (and folic acid versus placebo) in bipolar depression (CEQUEL): a 2×2 factorial randomised trial. Lancet Psychiatry 3 (1): 31–39.

227. Geddes, J.R., Calabrese, J.R., and Goodwin, G.M. (2009). Lamotrigine for treatment of bipolar depression: independent meta-analysis and meta-regression of individual patient data from five randomised trials. Br. J. Psychiatry 194 (1): 4–9.

228. Schoeyen, H.K., Kessler, U., Andreassen, O.A. et al. (2015). Treatment-resistant bipolar depression: a randomized controlled trial of electro-convulsive therapy versus algorithm-based pharmacological treatment. Am. J. Psychiatry 172 (1): 41–51.

229. Solomon, D.A., Keitner, G.I., Miller, I.W. et al. (1995). Course of illness and maintenance treatments for patients with bipolar disorder. J. Clin. Psychiatry 56 (1): 5–13.

230. Pallaskorpi, S., Suominen, K., Ketokivi, M. et al. (2015). Five-year outcome of bipolar I and II disorders: findings of the Jorvi bipolar study. Bipolar Disord. 17 (4): 363–374.

231. Perlis, R.H., Ostacher, M.J., Patel, J.K. et al. (2006). Predictors of recurrence in bipolar disorder: primary outcomes from the systematic treatment enhancement program for bipolar disorder (STEP-BD). Am. J. Psychiatry 163 (2): 217–224.

232. Angst, J. and Sellaro, R. (2000). Historical perspectives and natural history of bipolar disorder. Biol. Psychiatry 48 (6): 445–457.

233. Benard, V., Vaiva, G., Masson, M., and Geoffroy, P.A. (2016). Lithium and suicide prevention in bipolar disorder. Encephale 42 (3): 234–241.

234. Young, A.H. (2014). Lithium and suicide. Lancet Psychiatry 1 (6): 483–484.

235. Vieta, E., Günther, O., Locklear, J. et al. (2011). Effectiveness of psychotropic medications in the maintenance phase of bipolar disorder: a meta-analysis of randomized controlled trials. Int. J. Neuropsychopharmacol. 14 (8): 1029–1049.

236. Weisler, R.H., Nolen, W.A., Neijber, A. et al., Trial 144 Study Investigators. (2011). Continuation of quetiapine versus switching to placebo or lithium for maintenance treatment of bipolar I disorder (Trial 144: a randomized controlled study). J. Clin. Psychiatry 72 (11): 1452–1464.

237. Lähteenvuo, M., Tanskanen, A., Taipale, H. et al. (2018). Real-world effectiveness of pharmacologic treatments for the prevention of rehos-pitalization in a finnish nationwide cohort of patients with bipolar disorder. JAMA Psychiatry 75 (4): 347–355.

238. Altamura, A.C., Mundo, E., Dell'Osso, B. et al. (2008). Quetiapine and classical mood stabilizers in the long-term treatment of bipolar disorder: a 4-year follow-up naturalistic study. J. Affective Disord. 110 (1–2): 135–141.

239. Suppes, T., Vieta, E., Liu, S. et al., Trial 127 Investigators. (2009). Maintenance treatment for patients with bipolar I disorder: results from a north American study of quetiapine in combination with lithium or divalproex (trial 127). Am. J. Psychiatry 166 (4): 476–488.

240. Colom, F., Vieta, E., Sánchez-Moreno, J. et al. (2009). Group psychoeducation for stabilised bipolar disorders: 5-year outcome of a randomised clinical trial. Br. J. Psychiatry 194 (3): 260–265.

241. de Assis da Silva, R., Mograbi, D.C., LAS, S. et al. (2015). Insight across the different mood states of bipolar disorder. Psychiatr. Q. 86 (3): 395–405.

242. Murnane, E.L., Cosley, D., Chang, P. et al. (2016). Self-monitoring practices, attitudes, and needs of individuals with bipolar disorder: implications for the design of technologies to manage mental health. J. Am. Med. Inf. Assoc. 23 (3): 477–484.

243. Nicholas, J., Larsen, M.E., Proudfoot, J., and Christensen, H. (2015). Mobile apps for bipolar disorder: a systematic review of features and content quality. J. Med. Internet Res. 17 (8): e198.

244. Nutt, D.J. (2005). NICE: the National Institute of Clinical Excellence – or eccentricity? Reflections on the Z-drugs as hypnotics. J. Psychopharmacol (Oxford). 19 (2): 125–127.

245. Jones, I., Chandra, P.S., Dazzan, P., and Howard, L.M. (2014). Bipolar disorder, affective psychosis, and schizophrenia in pregnancy and the post-partum period. Lancet 384 (9956): 1789–1799.

246. Di Florio, A., Forty, L., Gordon-Smith, K. et al. (2013). Perinatal episodes across the mood disorder spectrum. JAMA Psychiatry 70 (2): 168–175.

247. Wesseloo, R., Kamperman, A.M., Munk-Olsen, T. et al. (2016). Risk of postpartum relapse in bipolar disorder and postpartum psychosis: a systematic review and meta-analysis. Am. J. Psychiatry 173 (2): 117–127.

248. Viguera, A.C., Whitfield, T., Baldessarini, R.J. et al. (2007). Risk of recurrence in women with bipolar disorder during pregnancy: prospective study of mood stabilizer discontinuation. Am. J. Psychiatry 164 (12): 1817–1824; quiz 1923.

249. Bergink, V., Bouvy, P.F., Vervoort, J.S.P. et al. (2012). Prevention of postpartum psychosis and mania in women at high risk. Am. J. Psychiatry 169 (6): 609–615.

250. McKnight, R.F., Adida, M., Budge, K. et al. (2012). Lithium toxicity profile: a systematic review and meta-analysis. Lancet 379 (9817): 721–728.

251. Cohen, L.S., Friedman, J.M., Jefferson, J.W. et al. (1994). A reevaluation of risk of in utero exposure to lithium. JAMA 271 (2): 146–150.

252. Kapfhammer, H.-P. and Lange, P. (2012). Suicidal and infanticidal risks in puerperal psychosis of an early onset. Neuropsychiatrie 26 (3): 129–138.

253. Vajda, F.J.E., O'Brien, T.J., Lander, C.M. et al. (2014). The teratogenicity of the newer antiepileptic drugs – an update. Acta Neurol. Scand. 130 (4): 234–238.

254. Dolk, H., Wang, H., Loane, M. et al. (2016). Lamotrigine use in pregnancy and risk of orofacial cleft and other congenital anomalies. Neurology 86 (18): 1716–1725.

255. Habermann, F., Fritzsche, J., Fuhlbrück, F. et al. (2013). Atypical antipsychotic drugs and pregnancy outcome: a prospective, cohort study. J. Clin. Psychopharmacol. 33 (4): 453–462.

256. Park, Y., Hernandez-Diaz, S., Bateman, B.T. et al. (2018). Continuation of atypical antipsychotic medication during early pregnancy and the risk of gestational diabetes. Am. J. Psychiatry 175 (6): 564–574.

257. Millan, M.J., Goodwin, G.M., Meyer-Lindenberg, A., and Ove Ögren, S. (2015). Learning from the past and looking to the future: emerging perspectives for improving the treatment of psychiatric disorders. Eur. Neuropsychopharmacol. 25 (5): 599–656.

258. Baldessarini, R.J. (2014). The impact of psychopharmacology on contemporary psychiatry. Can. J. Psychiatry 59 (8): 401–405.

259. Kandel, E.R. (1998). A new intellectual framework for psychiatry. Am. J. Psychiatry 155 (4): 457–469.

260. Stilo, S.A., Di Forti, M., Mondelli, V. et al. (2013). Social disadvantage: cause or consequence of impending psychosis? Schizophr. Bull. 39 (6): 1288–1295.

261. Trotta, A., Murray, R.M., and Fisher, H.L. (2015). The impact of childhood adversity on the persistence of psychotic symptoms: a systematic review and meta-analysis. Psychol. Med. 45 (12): 2481–2498.

262. Evans, M. (2016). The Making Room for Madness in Mental Health: The Psychoanalytic Understanding of Psychotic Communication, 1e, 240. Karnac Books.

263. Amick, H.R., Gartlehner, G., Gaynes, B.N. et al. (2015). Comparative benefits and harms of second generation antidepressants and cognitive behavioral therapies in initial treatment of major depressive disorder: systematic review and meta-analysis. BMJ 351: h6019.

264. Morrison, A.P., French, P., Stewart, S.L.K. et al. (2012). Early detection and intervention evaluation for people at risk of psychosis: multisite randomised controlled trial. BMJ 344: e2233.

265. Davies C, Radua J, Cipriani A, Stahl D, Provenzani U, Mcguire P, et al. (2018. b). Efficacy and acceptability of interventions for attenuated positive psychotic symptoms in individuals at clinical high risk of psychosis: a network meta-analysis. Front Psychiatry. 9:187. 10.3389/fpsyt.2018.00187

266. Davies, C., Cipriani, A., Ioannidis, J.P.A. et al. (2018). Lack of evidence to favor specific preventive interventions in psychosis: a network meta-analysis. World Psychiatry 17 (2): 196–209.

267. Jones, C., Hacker, D., Cormac, I. et al. (2012). Cognitive behaviour therapy versus other psychosocial treatments for schizophrenia. Cochrane Database Syst. Rev. 4 (Art. No.: CD008712). doi: https://doi.org/10.1002/14651858.CD008712.pub2.

268. Lynch, D., Laws, K.R., and McKenna, P.J. (2010). Cognitive behavioural therapy for major psychiatric disorder: does it really work? A meta-analytical review of well-controlled trials. Psychol. Med. 40 (1): 9–24.

269. Jauhar, S., McKenna, P.J., Radua, J. et al. (2014). Cognitive-behavioural therapy for the symptoms of schizophrenia: systematic review and meta-analysis with examination of potential bias. Br. J. Psychiatry 204 (1): 20–29.

270. Turner, D.T., van der Gaag, M., Karyotaki, E., and Cuijpers, P. (2014). Psychological interventions for psychosis: a meta-analysis of comparative outcome studies. Am. J. Psychiatry 171 (5): 523–538.

271. Guo, Z.-H., Li, Z.-J., Ma, Y. et al. (2017). Brief cognitive-behavioural therapy for patients in the community with schizophrenia: randomised controlled trial in Beijing, China. Br. J. Psychiatry 210 (3): 223–229.

272. Bird, V., Premkumar, P., Kendall, T. et al. (2010). Early intervention services, cognitive-behavioural therapy and family intervention in early psychosis: systematic review. Br. J. Psychiatry 197 (5): 350–356.

273. Garety, P.A., Fowler, D.G., Freeman, D. et al. (2008). Cognitive – behavioural therapy and family intervention for relapse prevention and symptom reduction in psychosis: randomised controlled trial. Br. J. Psychiatry 192 (6): 412–423.

274. Meyer, T.D. and Hautzinger, M. (2012). Cognitive behaviour therapy and supportive therapy for bipolar disorders: relapse rates for treatment period and 2-year follow-up. Psychol. Med. 42 (7): 1429–1439.

275. Scott, J., Paykel, E., Morriss, R. et al. (2006). Cognitive-behavioural therapy for severe and recurrent bipolar disorders: randomised controlled trial. Br. J. Psychiatry 188: 313–320.

276. Morrison, A.P., Pyle, M., Gumley, A. et al. (2018). Cognitive behavioural therapy in clozapine-resistant schizophrenia (FOCUS): an assessor-blinded, randomised controlled trial. Lancet Psychiatry 5 (8): 633–643.

277. Soo, S.A., Zhang, Z.W., Khong, S.J. et al. (2018). Randomized controlled trials of psychoeducation modalities in the management of bipolar disorder: a systematic review. J. Clin. Psychiatry 79 (3).

278. Pitschel-Walz, G., Leucht, S., Bäuml, J. et al. (2001). The effect of family interventions on relapse and rehospitalization in schizophrenia – a meta-analysis. Schizophr. Bull. 27 (1): 73–92.

279. Wykes, T., Huddy, V., Cellard, C. et al. (2011). A meta-analysis of cognitive remediation for schizophrenia: methodology and effect sizes. Am. J. Psychiatry 168 (5): 472–485.

280. Leff, J., Williams, G., Huckvale, M.A. et al. (2013). Computer-assisted therapy for medication-resistant auditory hallucinations: proof-of-concept study. Br. J. Psychiatry 202: 428–433.

281. Craig, T.K., Rus-Calafell, M., Ward, T. et al. (2018). AVATAR therapy for auditory verbal hallucinations in people with psychosis: a single-blind, randomised controlled trial. Lancet Psychiatry 5 (1): 31–40.

282. Razzaque, R. and Wood, L. (2015). Open dialogue and its relevance to the NHS: opinions of NHS staff and service users. Community Ment. Health J. 51 (8): 931–938.

283. Bergström, T., Seikkula, J., Alakare, B. et al. (2018). The family-oriented open dialogue approach in the treatment of first-episode psychosis: nineteen-year outcomes. Psychiatry Res. 270: 168–175.

284. Freeman, A.M., Tribe, R.H., Stott, J.C.H., and Pilling, S. (2018). Open dialogue: a review of the evidence. Psychiatr. Serv.; appips201800236.

285. Turkington, D. and Lebert, L. (2017). Psychological treatments for schizophrenia spectrum disorder: what is around the corner? BJPsych Adv. 23 (1): 16–23.

286. Leichsenring, F. and Steinert, C. (2017). Is cognitive behavioral therapy the gold standard for psychotherapy?: the need for plurality in treatment and research. JAMA 318 (14): 1323–1324.

287. Vandenberghe, F., Gholam-Rezaee, M., Saigí-Morgui, N. et al. (2015). Importance of early weight changes to predict long-term weight gain during psychotropic drug treatment. J. Clin. Psychiatry 76 (11): e1417–e1423.

288. Pérez-Iglesias, R., Martínez-García, O., Pardo-Garcia, G. et al. (2014). Course of weight gain and metabolic abnormalities in first treated episode of psychosis: the first year is a critical period for development of cardiovascular risk factors. Int. J. Neuropsychopharmacol. 17 (1): 41–51.

289. Shams, T.A. and Müller, D.J. (2014). Antipsychotic induced weight gain: genetics, epigenetics, and biomarkers reviewed. Curr. Psychiatry Rep. 16 (10): 473.

290. He, M., Deng, C., and Huang, X.-F. (2013). The role of hypothalamic H1 receptor antagonism in antipsychotic-induced weight gain. CNS Drugs 27 (6): 423–434.

291. Alvarez-Jiménez, M., González-Blanch, C., Vázquez-Barquero, J.L. et al. (2006). Attenuation of antipsychotic-induced weight gain with early behavioral intervention in drug-naive first-episode psychosis patients: a randomized controlled trial. J. Clin. Psychiatry 67 (8): 1253–1260.

292. Caemmerer, J., Correll, C.U., and Maayan, L. (2012). Acute and maintenance effects of non-pharmacologic interventions for antipsychotic associated weight gain and metabolic abnormalities: a meta-analytic comparison of randomized controlled trials. Schizophr. Res. 140 (1–3): 159–168.

293. Gaughran, F. and Lally, J. (2013). Non-pharmacological interventions reduce antipsychotic-associated weight gain in outpatients. Evid. Based Ment. Health 16 (1): 18.

294. Weiden, P.J. (2007). Switching antipsychotics as a treatment strategy for antipsychotic-induced weight gain and dyslipidemia. J. Clin. Psychiatry 68 (Suppl 4): 34–39.

295. Fleischhacker, W.W., Heikkinen, M.E., Olié, J.-P. et al. (2010). Effects of adjunctive treatment with aripiprazole on body weight and clinical efficacy in schizophrenia patients treated with clozapine: a randomized, double-blind, placebo-controlled trial. Int. J. Neuropsychopharmacol. 13 (8): 1115–1125.

296. Zheng, W., Li, X.-B., Tang, Y.-L. et al. (2015). Metformin for weight gain and metabolic abnormalities associated with antipsychotic treatment: meta-analysis of randomized placebo-controlled trials. J. Clin. Psychopharmacol. 35 (5): 499–509.

297. Liang, H., Li, H., Hu, Y. et al. (2016). Effects of topiramate for atypical antipsychotic-induced body weight gain and metabolic adversities: a systematic review and meta-analysis. Zhonghua Yi Xue Za Zhi 96 (3): 216–223.

298. Joffe, G., Takala, P., Tchoukhine, E. et al. (2008). Orlistat in clozapine- or olanzapine-treated patients with overweight or obesity: a 16-week randomized, double-blind, placebo-controlled trial. J. Clin. Psychiatry 69 (5): 706–711.

299. Siskind, D., Hahn, M., Correll, C.U. et al. (2019). Glucagon-like peptide-1 receptor agonists for antipsychotic-associated cardio-metabolic risk factors: a systematic review and individual participant data meta-analysis. Diabetes Obes. Metab. 21 (2): 293–302.

300. Singh, S., Chang, H.-Y., Richards, T.M. et al. (2013). Glucagonlike peptide 1-based therapies and risk of hospitalization for acute pancreatitis in type 2 diabetes mellitus: a population-based matched case-control study. JAMA Intern. Med. 173 (7): 534–539.

301. Monami, M., Nreu, B., Scatena, A. et al. (2017). Safety issues with glucagon-like peptide-1 receptor agonists (pancreatitis, pancreatic cancer and cholelithiasis): data from randomized controlled trials. Diabetes Obes. Metab. 19 (9): 1233–1241.

302. Hernandez, A.F., Green, J.B., Janmohamed, S. et al. (2018). Albiglutide and cardiovascular outcomes in patients with type 2 diabetes and cardiovascular disease (harmony outcomes): a double-blind, randomised placebo-controlled trial. Lancet 392 (10157): 1519–1529.

303. Pillinger, T., Beck, K., Gobjila, C. et al. (2017). Impaired glucose homeostasis in first-episode schizophrenia: a systematic review and meta-analysis. JAMA Psychiatry [cited 2017 Jan 16]; Available from: http://jamanetwork.com/journals/jamapsychiatry/fullarticle/2597705.

304. Lopez Vicchi, F., Luque, G.M., Brie, B. et al. (2016). Dopaminergic drugs in type 2 diabetes and glucose homeostasis. Pharmacol. Res. 109: 74–80.

305. Jesus, C., Jesus, I., and Agius, M. (2015). What evidence is there to show which antipsychotics are more diabetogenic than others? Psychiatr. Danub. 27 (Suppl 1): S423–S428.

306. Guenette, M.D., Hahn, M., Cohn, T.A. et al. (2013). Atypical antipsychotics and diabetic ketoacidosis: a review. Psychopharmacology (Berl). 226 (1): 1–12.

307. Lally, J., O' Loughlin, A., Stubbs, B. et al. (2018). Pharmacological management of diabetes in severe mental illness: a comprehensive clinical review of efficacy, safety and tolerability. Expert Rev. Clin. Pharmacol. 11 (4): 411–424.

308. Morrison, P.D. and Murray, R.M. (2009). From real-world events to psychosis: the emerging neuropharmacology of delusions. Schizophr. Bull. 35 (4): 668–674.

309. Goto, Y. and Grace, A.A. (2007). The dopamine system and the pathophysiology of schizophrenia: a basic science perspective. Int. Rev. Neurobiol. 78: 41–68.

310. Mace, S. and Taylor, D. (2015). Reducing the rates of prescribing high-dose antipsychotics and polypharmacy on psychiatric inpatient and intensive care units: results of a 6-year quality improvement programme. Ther. Adv. Psychopharmacol. 5 (1): 4–12.

311. Chang, A. and Fox, S.H. (2016). Psychosis in Parkinson's disease: epidemiology, pathophysiology, and management. Drugs 76 (11): 1093–1118.

312. Stahl, S.M. (2016). Mechanism of action of pimavanserin in Parkinson's disease psychosis: targeting serotonin 5HT2A and 5HT2C receptors. CNS Spectr. 21 (4): 271–275.

313. Cummings, J., Isaacson, S., Mills, R. et al. (2014). Pimavanserin for patients with Parkinson's disease psychosis: a randomised, placebo-controlled phase 3 trial. Lancet 383 (9916): 533–540.

314. Webster, P. (2018). Pimavanserin evaluated by the FDA. Lancet 391 (10132): 1762.

315. Woods, S.W., Morgenstern, H., Saksa, J.R. et al. (2010). Incidence of tardive dyskinesia with atypical versus conventional antipsychotic medications: a prospective cohort study. J. Clin. Psychiatry 71 (4): 463–474.

316. Peluso, M.J., Lewis, S.W., Barnes, T.R.E., and Jones, P.B. (2012). Extrapyramidal motor side-effects of first- and second-generation antipsychotic drugs. Br. J. Psychiatry 200 (5): 387–392.

317. Tamminga, C.A., Thaker, G.K., Moran, M. et al. (1994). Clozapine in tardive dyskinesia: observations from human and animal model studies. J. Clin. Psychiatry 55 (Suppl B): 102–106.

318. Spivak, B., Mester, R., Abesgaus, J. et al. (1997). Clozapine treatment for neuroleptic-induced tardive dyskinesia, parkinsonism, and chronic akathisia in schizophrenic patients. J. Clin. Psychiatry 58 (7): 318–322.

319. Stubbs, B., Gaughran, F., Mitchell, A.J. et al. (2015). Schizophrenia and the risk of fractures: a systematic review and comparative meta-analysis. Gen. Hosp. Psychiatry 37 (2): 126–133.

320. Raghuthaman, G., Venkateswaran, R., and Krishnadas, R. (2015). Adjunctive aripiprazole in risperidone-induced hyperprolactinaemia: double-blind, randomised, placebo-controlled trial. BJPsych Open 1 (2): 172–177.

321. Shim, J.-C., Shin, J.-G.K., Kelly, D.L. et al. (2007). Adjunctive treatment with a dopamine partial agonist, aripiprazole, for antipsychotic-induced hyperprolactinemia: a placebo-controlled trial. Am. J. Psychiatry 164 (9): 1404–1410.

322. Andersson, K.-E. (2011). Mechanisms of penile erection and basis for pharmacological treatment of erectile dysfunction. Pharmacol. Rev. 63 (4): 811–859.

323. Floody, O.R. (2014). Role of acetylcholine in control of sexual behavior of male and female mammals. Pharmacol. Biochem. Behav. 120: 50–56.

324. Olivier, B., Chan, J.S.W., Snoeren, E.M. et al. (2011). Differences in sexual behaviour in male and female rodents: role of serotonin. Curr. Top. Behav. Neurosci. 8: 15–36.

325. Dominguez, J.M. and Hull, E.M. (2005). Dopamine, the medial preoptic area, and male sexual behavior. Physiol. Behav. 86 (3): 356–368.

326. Baggaley, M. (2008). Sexual dysfunction in schizophrenia: focus on recent evidence. Hum. Psychopharmacol. 23 (3): 201–209.

327. Montejo-González, A.L., Llorca, G., Izquierdo, J.A. et al. (1997). SSRI-induced sexual dysfunction: fluoxetine, paroxetine, sertraline, and fluvoxamine in a prospective, multicenter, and descriptive clinical study of 344 patients. J. Sex Marital Ther. 23 (3): 176–194.

328. Nunes, L.V.A., Moreira, H.C., Razzouk, D. et al. (2012). Strategies for the treatment of antipsychotic-induced sexual dysfunction and/or hyperprolactinemia among patients of the schizophrenia spectrum: a review. J. Sex Marital Ther. 38 (3): 281–301.

329. Brown, D.A., Kyle, A., and Ferrill, M.J. (2009). Assessing the clinical efficacy of sildenafil for the treatment of female sexual dysfunction. Ann. Pharmacother. 43 (7): 1275–1285.

330. Rast, G. and Guth, B.D. (2014). Solubility assessment and on-line exposure confirmation in a patch-clamp assay for hERG (human ether-a-go-go-related gene) potassium channel inhibition. J. Pharmacol. Toxicol. Methods 70 (2): 182–187.

331. Perry, M.D., Ng, C.-A., Mann, S.A. et al. (2015). Getting to the heart of hERG K(+) channel gating. J. Physiol (Lond). 593 (12): 2575–2585.

332. Vandenberg, J.I., Perry, M.D., Perrin, M.J. et al. (2012). hERG K(+) channels: structure, function, and clinical significance. Physiol. Rev. 92 (3): 1393–1478.

333. Mizusawa, Y., Horie, M., and Wilde, A.A.M. (2014). Genetic and clinical advances in congenital long QT syndrome. Circ. J. 78 (12): 2827–2833.

334. Nielsen, J., Graff, C., Kanters, J.K. et al. (2011). Assessing QT interval prolongation and its associated risks with antipsychotics. CNS Drugs 25 (6): 473–490.

335. Cowan, J.C., Yusoff, K., Moore, M. et al. (1988). Importance of lead selection in QT interval measurement. Am. J. Cardiol. 61 (1): 83–87.

336. Lepeschkin, E. and Surawicz, B. (1952). The measurement of the Q-T interval of the electrocardiogram. Circulation 6 (3): 378–388.

337. Drew, B.J., Ackerman, M.J., Funk, M. et al. (2010). Prevention of torsade de pointes in hospital settings: a scientific statement from the American Heart Association and the American College of Cardiology Foundation. Circulation 121 (8): 1047–1060.

338. Davey, P. (2002). How to correct the QT interval for the effects of heart rate in clinical studies. J. Pharmacol. Toxicol. Methods 48 (1): 3–9.

339. Muzyk, A.J., Rayfield, A., Revollo, J.Y. et al. (2012). Examination of baseline risk factors for QTc interval prolongation in patients prescribed intravenous haloperidol. Drug Saf. 35 (7): 547–553.

340. Stein, L.I. and Test, M.A. (1980). Alternative to mental hospital treatment. I. Conceptual model, treatment program, and clinical evaluation. Arch. Gen. Psychiatry 37 (4): 392–397.

341. Cooper, B. (2010). British psychiatry and its discontents. J. R. Soc. Med. 103 (10): 397–402.

342. Yung, A.R., McGorry, P.D., McFarlane, C.A. et al. (1996). Monitoring and care of young people at incipient risk of psychosis. Schizophr. Bull. 22 (2): 283–303.

343. Fusar-Poli, P., Borgwardt, S., Bechdolf, A. et al. (2013). Psychosis high-risk state: a comprehensive state-of-the-art The review. JAMA Psychiatry 70 (1): 107–120.

344. Fusar-Poli, P., Cappucciati, M., Borgwardt, S. et al. (2016). Heterogeneity of psychosis risk within individuals at clinical high risk: a meta-analytical stratification. JAMA Psychiatry 73 (2): 113–120.

345. Fusar-Poli, P., Nelson, B., Valmaggia, L. et al. (2014). Comorbid depressive and anxiety disorders in 509 individuals with an at-risk mental state: impact on psychopathology and transition to psychosis. Schizophr. Bull. 40 (1): 120–131.

346. Lim, J., Rekhi, G., Rapisarda, A. et al. (2015). Impact of psychiatric comorbidity in individuals at ultra high risk of psychosis – findings from the longitudinal youth at risk study (LYRIKS). Schizophr. Res. 164 (1–3): 8–14.

347. Fusar-Poli, P., Bonoldi, I., Yung, A.R. et al. (2012). Predicting psychosis: meta-analysis of transition outcomes in individuals at high clinical risk. Arch. Gen. Psychiatry 69 (3): 220–229.

348. Hartmann, J.A., Yuen, H.P., McGorry, P.D. et al. (2016). Declining transition rates to psychotic disorder in "ultra-high risk" clients: investigation of a dilution effect. Schizophr. Res. 170 (1): 130–136.

349. van der Gaag, M., Nieman, D.H., Rietdijk, J. et al. (2012). Cognitive behavioral therapy for subjects at ultrahigh risk for developing psychosis: a randomized controlled clinical trial. Schizophr. Bull. 38 (6): 1180–1188.

350. Ising, H.K., Kraan, T.C., Rietdijk, J. et al. (2016). Four-year follow-up of cognitive behavioral therapy in persons at ultra-high risk for developing psychosis: the dutch early detection intervention evaluation (EDIE-NL) trial. Schizophr. Bull. 42 (5): 1243–1252.

351. Hutton, P. and Taylor, P.J. (2014). Cognitive behavioural therapy for psychosis prevention: a systematic review and meta-analysis. Psychol. Med. 44 (3): 449–468.

352. Stafford, M.R., Jackson, H., Mayo-Wilson, E. et al. (2013). Early interventions to prevent psychosis: systematic review and meta-analysis. BMJ 346: f185.

353. de Haan, L., Linszen, D.H., Lenior, M.E. et al. (2003). Duration of untreated psychosis and outcome of schizophrenia: delay in intensive psychosocial treatment versus delay in treatment with antipsychotic medication. Schizophr. Bull. 29 (2): 341–348.

354. Fraguas, D., Del Rey-Mejías, A., Moreno, C. et al. (2014). Duration of untreated psychosis predicts functional and clinical outcome in children and adolescents with first-episode psychosis: a 2-year longitudinal study. Schizophr. Res. 152 (1): 130–138.

355. Lappin, J.M., Morgan, K.D., Morgan, C. et al. (2007). Duration of untreated psychosis and neuropsychological function in first episode psychosis. Schizophr. Res. 95 (1–3): 103–110.

356. Craig, T.K.J., Garety, P., Power, P. et al. (2004). The Lambeth Early Onset (LEO) Team: randomised controlled trial of the effectiveness of specialised care for early psychosis. BMJ 329 (7474): 1067.

357. Craig, T., Fennig, S., Tanenberg-Karant, M., and Bromet, E.J. (1999). Six-month clinical status as a predictor of 24-month clinical outcome in first-admission patients with schizophrenia. Ann. Clin. Psychiatry 11 (4): 197–203.

358. Fusar-Poli, P., Díaz-Caneja, C.M., Patel, R. et al. (2016). Services for people at high risk improve outcomes in patients with first episode psychosis. Acta Psychiatr. Scand. 133 (1): 76–85.

359. McCrone, P., Craig, T.K.J., Power, P., and Garety, P.A. (2010). Cost-effectiveness of an early intervention service for people with psychosis. Br. J. Psychiatry 196 (5): 377–382.

360. Gafoor, R., Nitsch, D., McCrone, P. et al. (2010). Effect of early intervention on 5-year outcome in non-affective psychosis. Br. J. Psychiatry 196 (5): 372–376.

361. Bertelsen, M., Jeppesen, P., Petersen, L. et al. (2008). Five-year follow-up of a randomized multicenter trial of intensive early intervention vs standard treatment for patients with a first episode of psychotic illness: the OPUS trial. Arch. Gen. Psychiatry 65 (7): 762–771.

362. Rhodes, P. and Giles, S.J. (2014). "Risky business": a critical analysis of the role of crisis resolution and home treatment teams. J. Ment. Health 23 (3): 130–134.

363. Lelliott, P. (2006). Acute inpatient psychiatry in England: an old problem and a new priority. Epidemiol. Psichiatr. Soc. 15 (2): 91–94.

364. Tulloch, A.D., Khondoker, M.R., Thornicroft, G., and David, A.S. (2015). Home treatment teams and facilitated discharge from psychiatric hospital. Epidemiol. Psychiatr. Sci. 24 (5): 402–414.

365. Chang, W.C., Chan, G.H.K., Jim, O.T.T. et al. (2015). Optimal duration of an early intervention programme for first-episode psychosis: randomised controlled trial. Br. J. Psychiatry 206 (6): 492–500.

366. Slade, M. (2010). Mental illness and well-being: the central importance of positive psychology and recovery approaches. BMC Health Serv. Res. 10: 26.

367. Gilburt, H., Slade, M., Bird, V. et al. (2013). Promoting recovery-oriented practice in mental health services: a quasi-experimental mixed-methods study. BMC Psychiatry 13: 167.

368. Bellack, A.S. (2006). Scientific and consumer models of recovery in schizophrenia: concordance, contrasts, and implications. Schizophr. Bull. 32 (3): 432–442.

369. Fleischhacker, W.W., Arango, C., Arteel, P. et al. (2014). Schizophrenia – time to commit to policy change. Schizophr. Bull. 40 (Suppl 3): S165–S194.

370. Revier, C.J., Reininghaus, U., Dutta, R. et al. (2015). Ten-year outcomes of first-episode psychoses in the MRC ÆSOP-10 study. J. Nerv. Ment. Dis. 203 (5): 379–386.

371. Savill, M., Banks, C., Khanom, H., and Priebe, S. (2015). Do negative symptoms of schizophrenia change over time? A meta-analysis of longitudinal data. Psychol. Med. 45 (8): 1613–1627.

372. Killaspy, H. and Zis, P. (2013). Predictors of outcomes for users of mental health rehabilitation services: a 5-year retrospective cohort study in inner London, UK. Soc. Psychiatry Psychiatr. Epidemiol. 48 (6): 1005–1012.

373. Ramanuj, P.P., Carvalho, C.F.A., Harland, R. et al. (2015). Acute mental health service use by patients with severe mental illness after discharge to primary care in South London. J. Ment. Health 24 (4): 208–213.

374. Porter, M.E. (2010). What is value in health care? N. Engl. J. Med. 363 (26): 2477–2481.

375. Ray, J.C. and Kusumoto, F. (2016). The transition to value-based care. J. Interv. Card. Electrophysiol. 47 (1): 61–68.

376. Taylor, D.M., Sparshatt, A., O'Hagan, M., and Dzahini, O. (2016). Effect of paliperidone palmitate on hospitalisation in a naturalistic cohort – a four-year mirror image study. Eur. Psychiatry 37: 43–48.

377. McDaniel, R.R. (1997). Strategic leadership: a view from quantum and chaos theories. Health Care Manage. Rev. 22 (1): 21–37.

378. Marshall, D.A., Burgos-Liz, L., IJzerman, M.J. et al. (2015). Applying dynamic simulation modeling methods in health care delivery research-the SIMULATE checklist: report of the ISPOR simulation modeling emerging good practices task force. Value Health 18 (1): 5–16.

379. Sharp, L.F. and Priesmeyer, H.R. (1995). Tutorial: chaos theory – a primer for health care. Qual. Manage. Health Care 3 (4): 71–86.

380. Wise, J. (2014). Policeman tweets about 16 year old kept in cell because of lack of NHS beds. BMJ 349: g7408.

381. Keown, P., Weich, S., Bhui, K.S., and Scott, J. (2011). Association between provision of mental illness beds and rate of involuntary admissions in the NHS in England 1988–2008: ecological study. BMJ 343: d3736.

382. Higgins, J.P. (2002). Nonlinear systems in medicine. Yale J. Biol. Med. 75 (5–6): 247–260.

383. Kuziemsky, C. (2016). Decision-making in healthcare as a complex adaptive system. Healthcare Manage. Forum 29 (1): 4–7.

384. Peirce, J.C. (2000). The paradox of physicians and administrators in health care organizations. Health Care Manage. Rev. 25 (1): 7–28.

385. Bennett, C.C. and Hauser, K. (2013). Artificial intelligence framework for simulating clinical decision-making: a Markov decision process approach. Artif. Intell. Med. 57 (1): 9–19.

386. Stead, L.F., Perera, R., Bullen, C. et al. (2012). Nicotine replacement therapy for smoking cessation. Cochrane Database Syst. Rev. 11 (Art. No.: CD000146). DOI: 10.1002/14651858.

Index

Page numbers in **bold** indicate tables.

Advanced Prescribing in Psychosis, First Edition. Paul Morrison, David M. Taylor and Phillip McGuire.
© 2020 John Wiley & Sons Ltd. Published 2020 by John Wiley & Sons Ltd.